BE THE LEAST YOU CAN BE

Getting the Most Out of Your Phentermine Based Weight Loss Program

by

Dr. Mark Burtman

authorHOUSE®

AuthorHouse™
1663 Liberty Drive, Suite 200
Bloomington, IN 47403
www.authorhouse.com
Phone: 1-800-839-8640

© 2008 Dr. Mark Burtman. All rights reserved.

No part of this book may be reproduced, stored in a retrieval system, or transmitted by any means without the written permission of the author.

First published by AuthorHouse 7/21/2008

ISBN: 978-1-4389-0354-5 (sc)

Library of Congress Control Number: 2008906398

Printed in the United States of America
Bloomington, Indiana

This book is printed on acid-free paper.

TABLE OF CONTENT

1. Losing Weight by the Burtman Method — 1
2. Survival of the Fattest — 9
3. All Calories are not Created Equally — 17
4. Maintaining a Low-Carb diet in a High-Carb World — 25
5. Weight-loss Medications — 35
6. Misleading Labeling — 55
7. Natural is Not Necessarily Better — 65
8. Living by the Method — 73
9. Other Weight Loss Programs — 81
10. BurtmanWeightloss.com — 87
11. The Burtman Method of Losing Weight in a Nutshell — 97

1

Losing Weight by the Burtman Method

Welcome to page 1! The fact that you are here means that you've opened the book. That's good, because that implies that you are interested in doing something about your weight. Believe me, you're not alone. I also struggle with my weight, and it is through my own struggles that I have found a solution that works without making you miserable. That is why we are both here, you as the reader and myself as the author. If you are like me, you've tried several diets, supplements, and exercise programs, producing significant misery vastly out of proportion to the weight actually lost. I've been there waging war with my own self-control for several weeks only to lose a few pounds, which quickly return to my body within a few days of giving in to my desire to eat. Ultimately, we conclude that our efforts are fruitless, while our friends and loved-ones take cover against our moodiness in response to our feeble attempts at self-control.

I am not some fitness buff who spends every waking moment in the gym. Sure, I bought a Bowflex. One of these days I might even use it, but for now it's a great place to store books and discarded articles of clothing. You won't find me in tights aerobicizing to the oldies. For the most part, I'm just a guy with a weight problem just like you. Therefore, I can relate to you and your problem. I mean you can watch Suzanne Somers fitness videos, but Suzanne has never had a weight problem. How much would you ladies give to fit into the largest dress size that she ever ballooned into? The point is that we have a habitually beautiful, fit, and trim lady telling you how to lose weight. What does she know about having a weight problem? She's inherently slender. We are not. I think her solution to your problem is to never get overweight in the first place. That's fine for someone who needs to lose 5 or 10 quick pounds after a holiday food binge, but she's not going to transform you into a completely different physique. After you read this book and lose the weight that you want to lose, go ahead and watch her videos. I'm sure she will help you maintain that great figure. In the meantime, let me work with you as a fellow person who has struggled with his weight; as a person who understands what it is to have a busy schedule that interferes with our efforts to get some exercise. I know what it is to pay hundreds of dollars to join a fitness club and never go. I'm not in some ivory tower looking down on all you fat people while pretending to have all the answers to being thin despite the fact that I've never had a weight problem, could probably eat anything I desired and have no worries about weight gain. Don't you just despise those people? Let's call them the despicably thin. We'll deal with them later.

If you're still reading, you're probably wondering just who I am. Having a weight problem in and of itself is certainly no great qualification to help you lose weight. It's my own solution to the problem and the problems of many others that qualify me, and it doesn't require Richard Simmons like devotion to exercise and spandex.

I am not a dietician or exercise physiologist. I have no specified training in these subjects. Instead I am a physician specializing in Obstetrics and Gynecology. In medical school my training in nutrition was limited to what we had to learn in Biochemistry and Pathology. In biochemistry we learned the molecular function of carbohydrates, lipids, proteins, amino acids, and various cofactors and minerals. In Pathology we learned the diseases that occurred when there were deficiencies of the aforementioned nutrients. In clinical medicine we learned a little about how to prepare IV feeds including basic things like how many calories per gram of fat, carbohydrate or protein. That's it. I have no more training in the field of nutrition than any other physician. But I know enough to be effective. Soon you will too. In fact, in the absence of my own problems with my weight, I doubt that I would have ever ventured to write a book on this subject. Thus, it's really my personal interest in this subject that has driven me to this point.

It was the November 2003. I weighed 245 pounds at a height of 5'11" as my 40th birthday approached. I had Adult Onset Diabetes, and I was taking three different medications to marginally control my blood sugars. I ate whatever I wanted, which included most things that were off limits to diabetics, and I didn't exercise. I admit it; doctors make the worst patients. As my 40th birthday loomed large, I began to notice heart palpitations. I also made another observation in my own patients. I had patients of all sizes and shapes, but I rarely saw patients over the age of 75 who were significantly obese. That implied that they had died or were in no shape to venture out to my clinic, because they were bed-ridden or confined to a nursing home. The ones who were driving themselves, going to church, living alone, etc. were well under 200 pounds. I realized that if I wanted to live past the age of 80, I needed to get my weight down. Furthermore, the time to concern myself with living into my 80's was not when I hit my 70's. No, if I wanted to make it to the 80's, I needed to implement changes in my lifestyle now, before the damage was done. It was time to do something.

Okay, like most people with a vice the first step is to admit you have a problem. I like to eat. I admit it. Most people have some vice. For some its alcohol, others illicit drugs, smoking or various activities. I once asked a pregnant patient if she had quit smoking yet. She replied, "No, have you quit eating donuts?"

She had me there. I am well aware that my intake of sweets is as likely to kill me as someone else's cigarettes. Hence, we must approach my predilection to eat a dozen donuts in one sitting as an addiction like any other, whether it be smoking, drugs or alcohol. So, what's the prevailing to recommendation given to addicts? Quit completely. We don't advise cocaine addicts to limit their cocaine use to once a week. It's a strategy based on complete abstinence. So what about those of us who eat too much? Do we instruct those who overeat to give up food completely? Obviously not. Eating is the one vice that is actually essential to life. We can't completely avoid food in the same way that we can avoid drugs, alcohol and cigarettes. We have to eat or we die. Hunger is a survival mechanism. Thus, we have to face our vice each and every day and determine a way to moderate rather than completely eliminate the vice from our day to day life, which can result in a far more formidable challenge.

It wasn't the first time I had taken the challenge to eat better and lose weight. I had struggled with my weight for the last 20 years. But this time I wasn't feeling up to the challenge. I was tired of struggling with self-deprivation while getting nowhere. It was time to get some help. I had dabbled in writing prescription medications for weight loss for others. I did it begrudgingly, because I really didn't want to get involved in the field, especially in light of recent controversies surrounding the use of weight loss medications. However, one of my lady-friends had prevailed on me to help her with medications. But this time I went one step further. Instead of just writing one medication for her. I combined two medications, and I instructed her on a low carbohydrate diet. I had not previously formulated the concept of this triple therapy until she asked me for my help. Then the light bulb went on in my head— I had three modalities working synergistically to optimize the results. I had tried the diet. I had tried one of the medications before, but I had never until now seen all three methods employed at once. This combination produced rapid, profound results. I had happened upon a blockbuster method to effect weight loss. My friend went from 198 to about 165 in about 4 months.

Now face to face with my own mortality. It was time to dwell on my own weight problems. It was only a few months since my friend had lost her 30+ pounds. I thought of the Biblical passage in which Jesus alluded to the proverb which said, "Physician, heal thyself."(Luke

4:23) It was time to do just that. I would get a dose of my own medicine.

So I began at 245 pounds the same week as Thanksgiving. I chose the holidays to start, a time notorious for gluttony and expanding waistlines. In as much as I hoped that I would never see the topside of 240 pounds ever again, I took pictures of myself in nothing but gym shorts. In the back of mind, I considered that I might just be on to something significant. I decided then that if I succeeded, I would share my success with others. A picture at the start of my program would definitely capture the essence of my success. So, the Monday before Thanksgiving I took my first pills, and I was officially using the Burtman Method of Weight Loss. I am here to tell you that the effects were almost instantaneous. On the very first day, I cut my food intake by over 50% without any struggles with my will power. My blood sugar plummeted with the first dose to the point that I would actually bottom out. Eventually I was able to cut my blood sugar medicines to just one medication. During the first week from Monday to Monday, a week which included Thanksgiving, I lost 7 pounds. And, best of all, there was absolutely no struggle. My only concern was why I allowed myself to wait so long to initiate the therapy.

By the time I turned 40 I had lost about 30 pounds. I weighed less on my 40th birthday than I did on my 30th. I felt great, and now I was ready to solicit patients specifically for weight management. I took out an ad in the phone book, which brought me many patients. Then I became the beneficiary of the best kind of advertising: Word of mouth. In fact, it was better than word of mouth. It was like my patients were a walking billboard. The signs of weight loss would be on display in a matter of weeks from the first appointment. People would notice the thinning in the face, less belly hanging over the belt-line, and finally the loosening of once tight clothing. Before long, their friends and other family members were there to also seek my treatment as well.

I have patients losing in excess of 40 pounds with regularity, and it is not uncommon to see patients lose over 60 pounds in 5-6 months. Gone are the days of self-loathing over hours of exercise, Weight-Watcher meetings, which might produce a pound or two a week of weight loss. What I have stumbled upon is a program that produces profound, rapid results with minimal effort, and absolutely no misery. And best of all, you don't have to send me hundreds of dollars for some secret formula or concoction. You don't have to sign up in some pyramid business scheme requiring you to sell a product by harassing your friends and family. All you have to do is read the book and then enlist the support of your local physician. Then simply implement the dietary changes I advise you to make, and you will lose the weight as well.

Does it sound too good to be true? It's not. Do I sound like an infomercial? Most likely and I apologize for that. These visits in my office account for over 50% of my total appointments a week. That's over 200 patients a month. (Actually I have revised the number of patient numbers as I have written and rewritten segments of this book. So the preceding numbers in the text are way too low. Now that we have launched Burtmanweightloss.com, that total now surpasses 400 patients in just a week during my busy weeks. Our most recent tabulation for just the office in February and March of 2008 was 1050 office visits for diet pills alone. That does not include the evening seminars that bring us an additional 100-350 patients a week.) Most patients pay cash for their visits, because insurance companies don't usually cover this type of service. I don't offer any money back guarantees, but I do guarantee this: No patient is going to pay $55 a month to see me for my advice if they don't feel that they are improving. They are seeing me because their needs are being met. However, I will say this. I don't offer magic bullets. There is no medication that allows you to eat donuts and lose 50 pounds. Believe me, if there was such a thing, I'd be writing a best seller right now titled, Dr Burtman's Donut Diet Handbook, and I'd probably buy a chain of donut shops to go with it. This program is designed to help you help yourself, to help you actually get something out of your hard work to lose weight. The more good things you do to drive your weight down, the better your results. Patient's who come in expecting to not have to change the way they eat will be disappointed. The point of the book is that medicine can help you make those necessary changes without feeling like you're in a Turkish prison. So, let's lose some weight. If I can do it, you can do it too.

2

Survival of the Fattest

We were bred to be fat. It's really that simple. This may be the result of a 'Little Ice Age' that occurred between 1560 and 1850. There is considerable evidence that the global climate cooled significantly over that time. Cooler temperatures resulted in shorter growing seasons and failed crops, resulting in starvation, death, and disease. This resulted in massive upheaval throughout Northern Europe, which greatly affected the development of American colonization and immigration. Food shortages gave rise to the riots that spawned the French Revolution. Marie Antionette's famous words, "Let them eat cake," cost her her head at the guillotine. It was considered a callous comment about the starvation of peasants. The French revolution gave Napoleon an opportunity to ascend to power in France. He attacked Russia only to be defeated not by the Russian army; rather, it was the Russian winter that destroyed Napoleon's army, the majority dying of either exposure or starvation. Then there was the potato famine of Ireland from 1845-1849 that drove the Irish onto ships headed for America. The fact is that all American families have had something in their ancestry to drive them or force them from their ancestral homes with the common denominator of starvation playing a role either on the ships that brought them or conditions that forced them out of their country of origin. And guess who survived—the fat people. The skinny people who make aerobics videos now died. So, when you struggle to lose weight despite your best efforts to curb your intake, remember that you are a product of your breeding, which had to adapt to meager supplies of food. Thus you grow fat, because your ancestors survived.

Survival of the fittest is a concept that is attributed to Charles Darwin as an explanation for how and why various species have evolved over time. Whether or not you believe in the summation of these theories as it relates to the overall theory of evolution, this particular concept is not in dispute. It's a very simple fact that those who are strongest are most likely to survive. This gives rise to another concept called natural selection, in which nature naturally selects those who are the strongest by killing off the frail weaklings. In this way, only those strong enough to prevail against certain environmental hardships reach adulthood and have a chance to mate and reproduce. So, the fittest grow up, have sex, and reproduce their more durable traits, while the weak die, taking their weak genes with them to the grave.

As humans, we face the same obstacles within our own environment. However, our progression as a technological society has certainly minimized the impact of our environment on our survival. Hence, we are now able to breed generations of weaklings, as nearly all get to grow up to adulthood and breed, propagating their sniveling, little weak genes. But it wasn't always that way. In fact, it's only been that way for most humans for less than 100 years. For our forefathers and mothers, each and every year brought with it unique struggles, in particular, the struggle to assemble adequate food. If you are of European descent, it was long cold winters that drove the weak to their graves. If you are of African descent, it was the long periods of drought or famine that ravaged the land. Seafaring people could be lost at sea for prolonged periods of time. People of all races have had to adapt to prolonged periods of starvation, whether environmentally derived or endured as a byproduct of human conflict and cruelty. So, what is our primary mechanism to endure such hardships? It's fat.

Fat is a survival mechanism. During times of plenty humans partake of generous helpings of food. Whatever they do not need to burn immediately is stored for later use in the form of fat. Those with highly efficient metabolisms have more leftover calories, which can be converted to body fat for later use. Those are the people we see today as obese; however, in times past they were the ones best able to survive the long winters, droughts, and times of human cruelty. The despicably thin people who we now resent and envy for their perfect bodies simply died of starvation. So, when we lament how difficult it is to lose weight, it is necessary to remember that we, the fat, represent the survivors who shaped the evolution of our species. And when we try to force ourselves to lose weight, we are not simply fighting our own willpower. We are fighting the thousands of years of natural selection and adaptation that allowed our kind to endure many hardships. Simply stated, our body is designed to fight every effort we make to lose weight. Your body treats dieting like a death-threat, and will do all that it can to thwart your efforts. Consciously depriving yourself of food is not much different than depriving your body of sleep, water or air.

Modern day America provides a continuous plethora of food. Even though we consciously know that we should limit our food intake or grow fatter by the day, our primitive instincts, which guide our desires to eat, drink, sleep, and breathe, are completely oblivious to this fact. Our appetites are driven not only by a lack of food; they are also driven by the availability of food. Stroll past a restaurant and catch the aroma of what's being prepared inside, and suddenly your mouth may begin to water. Hunger pains may strike even though you may not have been giving food the least bit of thought until you actually came face to face with the appetizing odors. Again, this is an adaptation to the inconsistent availability of food that our ancestors contended with for many centuries. When food was available then, it behooved our forefathers and mothers to eat then and there, because food was not as likely to be available later. So, appetizing sensations are instinctively difficult to resist. This phenomenon is used against us daily by advertisers and purveyors of food. The TV is replete with ads that depict delectable treats, all of which set in motion actual reflexes that are difficult to thwart. The next thing you know, you're heading to the refrigerator in search of something to satisfy your newfound hunger.

But let's suppose that you have the willpower to withstand these instinctual desires to overeat. Perhaps you've affixed an "oink-oink" sound device to your refrigerator door or you have found some other way to overcome the urge to eat. Your body is still prepared for the self-imposed starvation that lies ahead. Remember, you are the product of generations of people who were specially adapted to withstand starvation. Step one was to eat plenty when food was available. Step two was to convert the extra food into body-fat. Now your low-calorie diet induces your body to activate step three: starvation mode. Again your body treats your dieting like an attack. It has no idea that this is intentional. Your body's instincts take over, viewing your self-imposed starvation as an attack, no different than an attack by wild beasts. To counteract this attack your body goes into a calorie conservation mode not unlike the hibernation mode that other animals take on. Your body will now fight to preserve calories, and your metabolism slows to a crawl. You may even notice that you become lethargic and disinterested in normal activities. You may become irritable like a hungry lion. Now you've created a situation that leaves you hungry and miserable only to find that your body fights to block your every effort by conserving calories. And you have your ancestors to thank that your body is so damn good at it.

This whole survival adaptation leaves you set up for the big disappointment at the end of the first week of misery. It's your first time back on the scale. Despite your misery, you're thrilled by your mind over body determination, which has effectively reduced your caloric intake. Now it's time to reap the reward and see how many pounds have melted away. Then you look in dismay at the numbers on the scale. You lost one pound. Now brokenhearted and demoralized, you drown your sorrows in a barrage of breadsticks and pizza, topped off by a hot fudge brownie sundae. By this time tomorrow you will not only gain back the weight you lost, but you will also pick up a few pounds, as your body is still in starvation mood. "What a close call!" your body thinks, "Another job well done. Better hang on to these extra calories. No telling when we'll have to survive something like that again."

Thus, losing weight is as much about overcoming years of evolution and basic survival instincts as it is about going on a diet. The goal of your body is to maintain its equilibrium. In order to lose weight, you must disrupt this equilibrium. In essence, you must shock the body by creating an unexpected imbalance. Whether it's calorie deprivation, as is attempted with dieting, or increasing caloric usage, as is attempted by increased exercise, your body will eventually adapt to it and find its equilibrium. Then the weight-loss will cease and your body will maintain the new status quo, attempting to rebuild the fat-stores that have been depleted by your determined efforts lose the weight at the first failure on your part to stick to your weight-loss program.

Dejected by your fruitless efforts to reclaim the physique of your youth, you may be wondering what's the point? How do I overcome this once essential survival mechanism? The answer is medication. Not medication alone: rather, medication in concert with your determined efforts to lose weight. The medication serves to nullify the body's survival mechanisms, which persistently thwart your attempts to really lose some weight. The medications are not there to allow you eat whatever you want and still lose weight. They simply interfere with the body's ability to maintain equilibrium when you do create the caloric imbalances. But the onus is still on you to create the decreased caloric input and the increased caloric output. The difference is that now you can see effective results quickly without permanently damaging your body's ability to survive times of hardship.

From here, this book will take you through my dietary strategy to not only reduce your calories, but to also choose the types of calories you take in, because all calories are not utilized equally. I will explain the pitfalls of traditional diets and why I feel that carbohydrates are the enemy of all attempts to lose weight. Then I will explain weight-loss medications, with descriptions of how they work and how they thwart your body's attempts to hang on to fat. I will go into carbohydrate content in various foods as well as strategies for staying low-carb in a high-carb society. Then I will finish with some pitfalls to beware of such as deceptive food labeling, which is designed to trick you into eating fattening foods. It's the wolf in sheep's clothing all over again.

3

All Calories are not Created Equally

The first question is what exactly is a calorie? The term calorie refers to a unit of energy just like dollars are a unit of money. In fact, your body handles calories in very much the same way you handle dollars. Energy can be stored or saved for later just like dollars can be saved in a bank. When your body saves calories it's in the form of fat. Unlike money, if your caloric savings account gets too big, it becomes a liability.

We get our calories by eating. There are 3 main forms of the calories we eat and then burn for energy. These include carbohydrates, fat, and protein. However, your body does not utilize these forms equally. If you eat a balanced diet, you will take in equal proportions of carbohydrates, fat, and protein. In such cases your body will utilize these calories in the most optimal way possible. That means that carbohydrates will be burned first for energy. Fat will be saved for later use and stored in unflattering ways on your body. Protein is used as the building blocks that make up your body. While your body can burn protein for energy, it will only do it as a last resort. Thus, the basis for low carbohydrate diets lies in the fact that you will never burn fat as long as you have carbohydrates in your system. But if you never eat carbohydrates, then you have no choice but to burn fats.

Think of carbohydrates as cash in your pocket. If you have a pocket full of cash, you do not go to the ATM and make a withdrawal. This is why it is virtually impossible to lose weight on a balanced or low-fat diet. There's no need to burn fat when carbohydrates are in good supply. Some are confused about these diets, because low carb diets tend to be high fat diets. How can you reduce the fat content of your body if you are eating more fat? To answer this we go back to the money analogy. Eating fat is like being paid with a check. If I write you a check, you cannot spend that check without cashing it. You can have a check in your pocket for thousands of dollars, but you will still need to go to the ATM if want to spend some cash. Going to the ATM reduces the amount of money in your bank account even if you have checks in your pocket. While the check in your pocket will eventually be deposited in your bank account, your body simply doesn't utilize fat the same way when there are no carbs on hand. So the key to losing weight is to eat an unbalanced diet. To do this we have to unlearn what we have been told for the last 50 years by dieticians, healthcare professionals, and exercise physiologists.

But before we can start a low-carb diet, we need to know what a carbohydrate actually is. It's important to be clear about that, because I have found that people get confused and before you know it, they're combining both a low-fat diet and a high-carb diet, which turns into a high-fat-high-carb diet, which is the worst diet to get on if you're trying to lose weight. In a word, carbohydrates are sugars. Carbohydrates come in two forms: simple and complex. Simple carbohydrates consist of one or two molecule carbohydrates. They tend to be sweet and tart. Most people will find these things easy to spot, because they taste like sugar should. Complex carbohydrates are not quite so obvious. These are known as starches. They don't taste like sugar. The most notable complex carbs are bread and potatoes, but cereals are also complex carbs. That's right, things like oatmeal and Special K are complex carbohydrates. The problem with complex carbs is that they have to be first broken down to simple carbs before they can be burned for energy. It's like eating an extended release carb. If you eat a meal rich in potatoes, breads, or cereals, it will be hours before you burn them up to the point that you will need to burn fat in order to sustain yourself. However, if you avoid carbohydrates all day long and then eat some simple carbs, your carb-starved body will rapidly burn these ready-to-use carbs, and you will be back to burning fat in short order. That means that you are better off eating something sweet instead of something starchy. So, a candy bar is preferable to eating a bowl of Special K. The key to that principle is that you must go without carbs all day and then finally treat yourself after a long period without carbs. Nibbling all day long is no different than eating an extended release complex carb. So it is better to eat the whole bag of M&M's at one time than to nibble on a few here and there throughout the day. Every time you take in some carbohydrates, you stop burning fat and revert to burning carbohydrates. So it is better to binge than to pace yourself, because the entire time between binges you will be burning fat.

So, how do we separate high carb foods from low carb foods? There is actually an easy way to separate the two groups of food. It has to do with what kingdom the food comes from. There's the plant kingdom and the animal kingdom. Almost all calories derived from the plant kingdom are carbohydrate. That includes both fruits and vegetables. You can get away with eating light, leafy, green vegetables, because they have very few carbs in them despite the fact that they get 100% of their calories from Carbohydrates. I call these light carbs. But just about everything else, including beans, nuts and soy products, are going to be full of carbs. About the only low carb fruit I know of is the avocado, which is the key ingredient of guacamole.

The animal kingdom is comprised mostly of fat and protein. Obviously, meat and seafood will consist almost exclusively of fat and protein. There are also animal byproducts to consider as well. Whole milk will have carbohydrate, fat and protein, but many milk products are low in carbohydrate. It's pretty easy to distinguish between hi-carb dairy products and low-carb dairy products. If it's sweet, like yogurt and ice cream, you can expect to find carbohydrate. If it's not sweet, like cheese, butter, and sour cream, you need not worry too much about blowing your low-carb diet on these foods. All eggs are low-carb. Then are varying combinations of these products, such as mayonnaise, margarine, and various oils. In fact, all oils are fats, though many oils may actually be derived from vegetables. This opens the door to tuna salad and chicken salad. Most dressings are also low carb. I also lump mushrooms in with the animal kingdom even though it's actually a fungus.

Using the above criteria it's pretty easy to distinguish between high and low carbohydrate foods, though it's certainly never a bad idea to read the label of the item in question to ascertain the actual carb content within the food. I'll go into reading labels more later. However, when you're in a restaurant, you won't have package labels to peruse as you make your selections. That's why I emphasize a more conceptual approach.

Having distinguished between low carb and high carb foods, I have now opened up the menu to items that are not normally associated with dieting and excluded others that you may have eaten in good conscience. For example, cereal is a very dense carb, so I discourage eating things like Special K, Granola, Raisin Bran, and oatmeal. Even if it's whole wheat bread, it's still a high carb grain that will shut off the fat burning process for the balance of the day. On the other hand, I am all in favor of eating fried chicken, Pizza(as long as it's thin crust), and a whole host of greasy foods. I eat at Pizza Hut's buffet at least once a week, and I encourage people to eat at KFC every day if they want to. "But isn't the breading carbohydrate?" I am asked repeatedly.

"Of course, it is," I reply, "but what do you normally eat when you go to KFC? It's not the breading on the chicken that packs the carbs into your blood stream. It's the mashed potatoes, the biscuits, the corn on the cob, the baked beans, and candied apples they add in as sides that constitute the majority of the meal. Stick to just the chicken, and you'll have a moderately low-carbohydrate meal."

It's not the Double Quarter with Cheese that gets you. It's the french fries, sugared soda, and milk shake that get you. Stick to the burger and you'll be cutting carbs. Get rid of the bun, and you'll lose even more carbs. Sometimes I'll take a few bites with the bun. Then once my hunger is abated, I finish off the rest of the burger without the bun. When it comes to bigger sandwiches, I'll use tortilla wraps as opposed to a large hoagie bun. I also like to take barbecue and eat it on a platter and then accompany that with some chicken tenders dipped in ranch. It's very filling and very little carb.

I often hear from my patients some excuse about being on the road and having to eat out a lot. That excuse doesn't hold water with me. I eat out almost every meal, especially now that I've taken my program on the road. Every restaurant in America has something on it that's low-carb. You just have to think outside the bun as they say in the Taco Bell ad. It's really thinking outside the french fry mentality that you grew up with that is essential.

Finally I want to emphasize that the carbs you drink count just as much as the carbs you eat. Many people drink a wide variety of sweet drinks ranging from sodas to juices, Gatorade, and sweet teas among others. The problem with drinking your calories is twofold. First, if you don't drink your calories, you can eat more. There's no point in trying to control your appetite, if you're going to bypass the whole strategy by drinking your calories. Secondly, every time you sip some sugar, what happens? You stop burning fat. Since you tend to drink throughout the day, you will never be without sugar long enough to be compelled to burn fat. In fact, if you consume sodas the way I do, you don't have to eat to meet your daily caloric requirements. You will not starve to death drinking Coke. You may die of other digestive tract maladies, but it won't be from a lack of calories. There are 140 calories in every can of Coke. A 24-ounce bottle has as many calories as a Milky Way Bar. If you drink ten cans a day, you will take in 1400 calories a day, all of which are carbohydrates that are consumed throughout the day. I still remember the week I switched to Diet Coke 20 years ago. I used what I call 'Twinkie Logic'. I realized that I could eat two more Twinkies a day and still lose weight by switching to Diet Coke, because I would still be cutting 1000 calories a day out of my diet. Sure enough, I lost 5 pounds the week I made the switch, and it was the last time I managed to get my weight below 200 pounds. The next year I got married and that was the last of my sub-200 pound years. So get rid of the sugared drinks, which is less complicated than getting rid of your spouse. If you don't like the taste of diet drinks, give it about two weeks and you'll never go back. The aftertaste will disappear. I promise you I enjoy my sugar free drinks just as much as you enjoy your regular drinks, only your indulgence comes at a cost of 1000 calories and mine is a complete freebie. To illustrate just how profoundly insensitive my taste buds are to the after taste of diet sodas, I have to have someone else taste my sodas for me at restaurants if I suspect that I have been given a regular, sugared Coke by mistake, because I can't use the aftertaste to distinguish between the two. Then I rely on some sugared soda junkie to do the tasting for me.

While we're on the topic of beverages, it seems appropriate to discuss the issue of alcohol. Alcohol itself is not a carbohydrate. In actuality, it's ethyl alcohol, which is not burned preferentially; rather, it is burned as a necessity to eliminate from your blood stream. My recommendation is to drink higher proof liquor with diet sodas or mixers. Alcohol is made when bacteria metabolize the carbohydrates into alcohol, so the higher the proof, the fewer the remaining carbohydrates. Thus, the lower the proof or sweeter the beverage the more the carbohydrate that is left for you to metabolize. Beer is notoriously bad, because it's only between 3% to 6% alcohol. The rest is water and carbohydrate. The other problem with beer is that it tends to be consumed in large quantities during football games, picnics, and parties. That's why we see beer-bellies. However, we usually don't see things like vodka-bellies, because it's a lot harder to consume 24 vodkas in a day, unless you're stuck in a Siberian Gulag. Most ladies I deal with on diet are likely to have one or two drinks as a nightcap or on a weekend. The carbs that are generally consumed in a sweeter beverage are simple carbs and therefore quickly metabolized. My opinion is that if you're drinking enough drinks to ruin your diet, you're probably drinking enough liquor to adversely affect your life too. So just drink moderately and everything should be fine.

4

MAINTAINING A LOW-CARB DIET IN A HIGH-CARB WORLD

This is the chapter where I give the details of my ideas regarding a low carbohydrate diet. I have no new insights about this diet that have not been said elsewhere. However, I hope to offer some ideas on surviving on this diet, and I hope to reiterate why I am such a proponent of this diet.

But before I go into the diet, let's go way back. I mean back to when it first started for you. You know, your addiction to carbohydrates, which has you reading this book in the first place. It all starts with your first meal. By first meal, I am not trying to get into any oedipal conflicts, as I am not referring breast milk or formula. Let's not go that far back. Instead, let's just go back as far as your first solid food. Do you remember it? Probably not, but I bet you can guess what it consisted of. It was most likely, unless you were raised by a pack of wolves, a meal consisting of pure carbohydrates. Perhaps it was baby cereal or some fruity sauce. The point is that it was a purely carbohydrate meal, and it was satisfying irrespective of whether your caretaker imitated an airplane coming in for a landing into your mouth. From there the addiction began to take hold.

Sugar and dough have wonderful properties in so far as they can be made to take on the shape of any super-hero, cartoon character, or latest star-fighter. Your earliest memories are probably composed of hours of television. After watching your favorite character save the universe, you then had the option of eating him or her for breakfast that morning. And if a certain cereal wasn't modeled after an existing cartoon character, they made one up like Captain Crunch, the Silly Rabbit, or Tony the Tiger. Soon each and every meal was laced with high fructose corn syrup derived flavors. So, your addiction to carbs began even before your earliest memories.

This addiction has been further reinforced by the anti-fat propaganda that you were force-fed in your health classes. Those were the same classes that introduced you to the four food groups and told you that you needed several helpings of carbohydrates a day. They didn't tell you some key things. First, your body has no trouble converting carbohydrate to fat. Second, your body will not burn fat as long as there is carbohydrate available in your system. The diet that you were instructed to follow virtually guarantees you that you will always have a steady supply of carbohydrate available to metabolize. Yes, the diet is an excellent way to prevent starvation. If you had been stranded high atop the Andes Mountains for one month with nothing to eat but fellow passengers, I would have highly recommend such a diet upon your return to the civilized world. However, we, who have already shown our innate abilities to survive starvation, will simply take this balanced (high-carb) diet as an excellent opportunity to produce more fat in anticipation of our own mountain-top ordeal. But these adventures are not a likely occurrence for us. Thus, we grow thicker by the year like rings on a tree.

Weight-loss is accomplished in many ways. You have also been told that it's a simple matter of calories. Take in more calories than you use, you get fatter. Use more calories than you consume, you lose weight. However, it's not that simple. As I said earlier, your body fights to keep your weight from dropping. Take in fewer calories, and your body finds a way to burn fewer of them. Just like when you're short of cash, you spend less. Take in more calories, then your body utilizes the excess as an opportunity to store up for future dieting attempts. Most classical weight-loss experts tell you that exercise is the key. It burns calories, and it does induce your body into burning more calories. So, the classic approach is to cut caloric intake through generalized calorie reduction, and increase calorie usage through high impact exercise. This approach can work wonderfully, but there are walls that can be difficult to overcome. If you have not exercised for a while, you may see a rapid response at first, maybe 5 pounds the very first week. However, once you hit a rhythm your body reequilibrates to your new routine, and suddenly the weight stops coming off. Your body tends to lose weight when it is caught off guard. Give it a week or two and it will figure out what you are up to, and find a way to return itself to normalcy. That's not to say that if you maintain the intense workout schedule that you have selected for yourself that you won't lose 30 pounds over the course of 6 to 24 months. But consider this, over the course of 24 months you will encounter 2 Christmases, 2 Thanksgivings, 2 birthdays, numerous invitations to weddings, graduation parties, funerals, and 100 Friday-evening happy-hours. Additionally, if you are woman with children, you will need to care for the children that caused you to gain weight, while serving them their cartoon character shaped, high carb treats. If you are a working mother, your day likely starts before 6 AM, and you will be on the move non-stop until at least 7 PM. Only then will you have time to exercise; however, by then you are more likely to just want to sit down and relax for the first time in 13 hours and watch CSI rather than attack a stair-master or aerobics work-out. You've probably tried all of this and become demoralized in the process, which is probably why you're reading this page right now. The point is the low-carb, high-intensity exercise program sounds great, but in reality it is a trifling experience to maintain unless you're a professional lifeguard, swimsuit model, or movie star. The purpose of this book is to help you find a less trifling way to lose the weight, something a super-mom can do.

Traditional weight-loss experts tell you to cut fat, and there are an abundance of 'fat-free' products on the market. But your body will have no trouble maintaining it's present weight even at a greatly reduced total caloric intake, as long as it receives adequate carbohydrates. You may not gain weight, but your bland baked potato without butter will keep your metabolism going for many hours. Ironically, if you ate a stick of butter or margarine the same size as the potato and nothing else, your body would be in a panic, because there would have been no carbohydrates available for immediate consumption. There is no chopped wood available for the fireplace, no cash in your metabolic pocket. Your body must chop more wood, or make a withdrawal from the fat bank. The mass of margarine does not get utilized effectively in the absence of carbohydrate, and you lose weight, as the body begins to break down the fat stores in your cells to maintain the metabolic fireplace. I am not telling you to eat straight margarine even though it will help you lose weight better than the potato. I am simply telling you that nothing induces fat burning better than depriving your body of carbohydrate.

Calorie counting is a frustrating and inferior way to lose pounds. If you eliminate carbohydrates, you will never have to count a calorie again. Eat when you're hungry and avoid carbohydrates and the weight will have to come off. Again, as I write this, it looks good on paper, but, alas, we did start out this chapter by saying we have an addiction to carbohydrates. You are never more reminded of this fact until you go a week without any carbohydrate at all. I've been there. You don't quite appreciate how satisfying the carbs are until you feel the constant hunger. Potatoes and breads are very satisfying, and I am telling you to give them up. But don't lose heart. I have a way to make this a pleasant and uplifting experience. If all I had to offer was the low-carb diet, I would never have written this book. Like I said earlier, there are wonderful books already written on the benefits and strategies of the low-carbohydrate diet. It's my ability to use medication with the diet that will make these benefits available to you, but you must read on to learn more about these medications.

But for now, back to the evil carbohydrates. Many authorities have replaced calorie counting with carbohydrate gram counting. I find that to be too much work. I have never counted my carb-grams, and I don't expect my patients to either. Thus, I am not going to present any recommendations regarding how many carbohydrate grams you should consume. I simply propose that you eat as few as you can stand. All carbohydrates that you take in should be accidental little carb grams that simply can't be eliminated, because they are a small component of what you are eating anyway. Having said that, let me introduce you to my own concept regarding carbohydrates. I prefer to use the terms dense carbs, simple carbs, and light carbs.

Dense carbs are composed of the complex carbohydrates also known as starches. As you may recall, these carbs are long chains of single molecules of glucose. These are the worst carbs. They are also the easiest to identify, and at times the hardest to avoid. They include breads, potatoes, corn, cereal, among other starchy things. They are the worst carbs to consume, because they are packed with sugar molecules, and they take time to break down once they are eaten. Thus a large baked potato can take the better part of the afternoon to break down into the simple sugar molecules that your body can actually metabolize. Therefore, you will not be burning any fat during that period of time.

Then there are the simple carbs. If it's sweet, it's simple. These are single or double molecules. These simple carbs are found in table sugar, fruits, and milk. Since these are simple molecules or double molecules, they can be quickly utilized. A lot of people think fruit is great for a diet. Certainly the vitamins that are found in fruit are quite beneficial, but the sugar is not. I've had patients come into my office confused as to why they don't lose weight. When I question them about their diet, they confidently reply that they eat fruit salad for lunch. While a single piece of fruit will not destroy your diet, a fruit salad will. In a fruit salad there are many fruits cut into pieces to create a concentrated sugar feeding frenzy. People have similar misconceptions about how healthy fruit juice is. To drink a glass of juice you must consume the sugar content of several pieces of fruit. There are also many who think that dried fruit is a healthy snack, but that's true only if you are striving to increase your sugar intake. The drying process simply eliminates the water content of the fruit. It does nothing to the sugar content, however, it makes the fruit less filling, so you can eat more of them, which means that you will consume more pieces of fruit than you normally would and therefore more sugar. Simple sugars are also what are used to sweeten beverages unless they are sugar free.

Nonetheless, if you are going to cheat with a carbohydrate, I am actually of the opinion that you are going to do less damage with the occasional candy bar than you would with a baked potato. In fact, I will admit to frequently eating sweets during my 35-pound plummet. Even though your mother and your dentist have always cautioned you about eating excessive sweets, I am telling you that a chocolate bar will do less to sabotage your efforts than a baked potato, an order of french fries or a bag of potato chips. Now, this is assuming that you have been diligently maintaining your low-carb diet. Perhaps you have chosen to reward yourself for good behavior. So, why is a candy bar the lesser of the two evils? The answer is because a candy bar is composed almost entirely of simple carbohydrates, whereas a potato product is composed entirely of complex carbohydrates. So, which one do you think will be used up the fastest? Remember, the complex carbohydrates have to be broken down first to its constituent parts, which are simple carbohydrates.

Thus it will take several hours to clear those carbs—to burn them up before your body resumes its task of burning fat. However, when you eat simple carbs after depriving your body of carbs for many hours, days or even weeks, your body will burn these simple carbs up quickly leaving no trace behind in a matter of a few hours. Regardless of which form of carbohydrate you take in, you will interrupt the process of breaking down and burning fat. So, the key is to choose the form of carbohydrate that is eliminated the fastest, which gets you back to the desired task of burning fat. While a one-time snack of candy will do less harm to your diet than a one time helping of potatoes, I must emphasize that this is not a license to graze on candy. If you eat candy all day, you essentially do the same thing that is accomplished by eating a loaded baked potato. In which case, you can forget about burning fat on that day.

While I'm on the topic of cheating, let me cover another issue along these lines. When you eat a low-carbohydrate diet, you will eat more fat as a percentage of calories in your total diet. As I said earlier, there are over 9 calories per gram of fat, which is almost triple the calories found in carbs. However, in the absence of an appropriate amount of carbohydrates that doesn't hold true. Fats are not well utilized in low-carb diets. A common failure in these diets is the impulsive carb-binge. Let's suppose you've been good all day. For lunch you had chicken salad. For supper you ate a steak and salad with creamy dressing. But you were still hungry, so you then ate some pork rinds with dip. You're still okay with the diet, but you've definitely piled on the fat. If you stop there, you'll be fine. But you're still having cravings. That's when you find the Girl Scout Cookies, and you eat the whole box. Once the craving is satisfied, your hunger is replaced by guilt. While I am not an advocate of feelings of guilt, I do acknowledge that your setback has served as a double whammy. Not only have you consumed a box full of carbs, you've added fuel to the fire by giving your body a huge supply of fat. Now that you have a ready supply of carbohydrates, the many grams of fat that you just ate will now be used for their intended purpose, to be stored as body fat. You will now realize the full impact of every calorie you have consumed.

Now I will define what I mean by light carbs. These are foods that are composed entirely of carbohydrate; however, they have so few calories that they can still be consumed on a low carb diet. Examples of these are light leafy green vegetables like lettuce, broccoli, and spinach. These vegetables are composed mostly of non-digestible carbs and water. Eating these types of vegetables will give you a small amount of carbohydrate without destroying your diet, which will help you moderate the amount of ketones that your body is producing.

Along that line of thinking I have another type of carbohydrate which I refer to as incidental carbs. These are carbohydrates that will sneak into your diet as an ingredient of your food. True low carb fanatics will even eliminate these carbs, but I believe you can still lose weight without going to that point. Nonetheless, if you can eliminate these carbs out of your diet, you will do even better. A perfect example of an incidental carb is lasagna. Lasagna is made of meat, sauce cheese and noodles. The sauce is based on tomatoes, which are carbohydrate. The noodles are based on grain, which are complex carbs. I believe that you can eat lasagna, because the carbohydrate component is the minority component of the dish, but they are present just the same. Another incidental carb is bread on sandwiches or burgers. Some people will peel the bread off of the sandwich. Hardees has introduced the low-carb burgers, which are wrapped in lettuce. If I get a sandwich, I will usually eat the bread, but I never get the fries. Still there are strategies to reduce the incidental carbs further. A lot of restaurants now use tortillas in place of buns to reduce carbs, but the tortillas are still primarily carbohydrate. If you are going to eat pizza, you can reduce your carbs by getting thin crust and then not eating the crust at all. There are also certain products that are often served as sandwiches, but can easily be eaten with the bread. Barbecued pork, chicken salad, and tuna salad are all examples. Barbecue sauce has some carbohydrate in it, but I'll still eat it. So does gravy along with the breading on fried chicken. I'll eat these incidental carbs, which will keep me out of ketoacidosis without destroying my diet. Of course, there is a fine line between eating incidental carbs and overdoing it with carbs, so be careful.

Now I've presented you with my diet. It's not hard to understand, but it can be hard to follow. That's where the medication comes in. The medication will make the diet an easy one to follow, and it will keep your body burning calories. The weight will begin to fall off like never before. The results will come quickly often within a few days. Like one of my patients said, "There is nothing more motivating than success."

Thus a positive cycle begins.

5

Weight-loss Medications

Medications can help you lose weight by three mechanisms of action. First, they may decrease one's appetite. This reduces calories taken in by causing you to crave less food. Second, they can help stimulate your metabolism to burn more calories. If you consume a higher percentage of the calories you eat via your metabolic machinery, then you'll have less left over to store as fat, or you'll be more likely to burn fat when your metabolic needs exceed your available caloric intake. Lastly, there are medications that may interfere with digestion itself, which will further reduce the calories available with a given meal. I believe that in order to have the most optimal medicinal program for weight-loss, you must have each of the aforementioned mechanisms at work. There are many medications available for assistance in weight-loss; however, there is no single medication that encompasses all three mechanisms of action. Thus, a combination of medications is required.

As I have looked around at the various regimens available for treatment of obesity, I have seen very little written about the use of combined treatment modalities. Everyone seems so intent on touting their own product as the best way to accomplish weight-loss. They offer no alternative or suggestion for combining their own method with others. I've had patients say, "No thanks, Dr. Burtman,

I want to try this or that program first and then I'll come to you if I need it."

They act as if it's an either-or proposition. It's not. My program is designed to help you get more out of any other program that you wish to try. In fact, let me emphasize now that my purpose is NOT to simply throw medication at you while you continue the same existence that brought to your present weight. This is NOT Dr Burtman's fabulous Doughnut Diet. It's much more about using these medications to help you beat your addiction to carbohydrates. Any other attempts to involve other programs of diet and exercise are not only encouraged but required. The difference is that by combining the medications and the programs already available you can lose those pounds in a matter of weeks and months rather than an entire year.

If you look at the data, most medications show statistically significant weight loss at as little as 2 pounds per month. That's only 24 pounds per year. Most people won't stick to anything with such slow results. I wouldn't be writing an average of 100-300 prescriptions a week for weight-loss pills if that's all I was able to accomplish. The reason I have so many patients now for weight-management is a direct relationship to significant amount of weight they are losing. I am striving to get my patients to lose 8-12 pounds per month. Some lose more and some lose less. Personally, I lost 18 pounds in my first month. I ended up losing 32 pounds before I stopped really trying. It took about 3 months. I have many patients who have lost over 40, and a few who have lost 60-70 pounds. There are some who have exceeded 100 pounds over the course of a few years. It's a function of effort and how much weight one needs to lose. I'll delve into those issues in more detail later.

It's time to meet my two favorite medications. The first one is the most effective weight-loss medication legally available today. It is Phentermine. Phentermine may sound familiar, either because it is probably the most widely prescribed diet pill in the U.S. today, or because it was one of the Phens of Fen-Fen fame. Phentermine is a type of amphetamine. Amphetamines are stimulants. They're also known as uppers. As stimulants, they are known to do two out of the three aforementioned mechanisms described above. The most obvious is that they stimulate the metabolism, so that you burn calories. Secondly, they will lower your appetite. They have other pleasant side-effects as well. In as much as they stimulate, they give a person energy and provide you with a very comforting sense of well-being and optimism without deluding you into thinking you can fly. It's easy to stay motivated while on the diet. Contrary to what people would assume, rather than make most people hyper, agitated and easily distracted, they tend to give people focus and the ability to concentrate. This is why Attention Deficit and Hyperactivity Disorder is treated with other medications in this class like Adderall and Ritalin.

I'll admit that I was not only hesitant to take Phentermine. I was also hesitant to prescribe these pills as well. However, since the Fen-Fen scare, there have been no major reported complications with the appropriate use of Phentermine. I was also worried that it would affect my judgment, temperament, and coordination. As a physician and surgeon, I could not afford to compromise any of those attributes. Fortunately, I have been most pleased with my behavior while on Phentermine. In fact, I have seen my energy and productivity increase as a result of my use of Phentermine, and it doesn't come to a screeching halt when I come off of the drug either. The fact that I have successfully overcome a significant problem keeps me pumped even during my break from the drug.

Nonetheless, as Phentermine is a stimulant, prolonged use can still put a strain on the heart, which can lead to damage of the heart valves. Most studies involving Fen-Fen showed heart valve disease at longer than 6 months. Therefore, I limit my patients to 6 months of therapy per year. Then they skip 6 months, after which I place them once again on the medicine if they still need it. So, I really push patients to get adjusted to the lower-carbohydrate diet while they are on the Phentermine. If the patient resumes the bad habits that caused the obesity to start with, then they will simply gain the weight back. Sometimes they will even exceed the weight that they started with. Hence, it takes a true commitment to change the way they eat, or the success will be temporary. Still, I do expect that everyone, myself included, will gain some of the weight back. My goal is to make it less than 10 pounds, so that they can quickly get that weight off when they come back and start losing more soon after they resume taking the Phentermine.

So, I have my patients use the appetite suppressant qualities of Phentermine to facilitate their strict adherence to a low carbohydrate diet. Without significant hunger the diet becomes easy to maintain. There will still be hunger, but it is easily satisfied without needing to stuff bread and potato products into one's belly. Then by the time the 6 months are up, it is my goal that a patient has adjusted to the diet, so that he or she can maintain it to some degree while they take a break from the medicine.

As you get further into the regimen of taking the Phentermine, the hunger may become more noticeable. However, the Phentermine still stimulates the metabolism. Thus I still encourage people to continue even if there is more hunger. I liken the calorie burning phenomenon to placing you on a metabolic treadmill. Without actually doing experiments, I actually believe that the increased calorie burning can equate to burning the same amount of calories as an exercise program without actually doing the exercise. Interestingly, your body can adapt to a program of exercise, especially one that can involve establishing a pace, like jogging. If you suddenly start jogging 5 miles a day, you will lose weight for the first week or two, but then you will hit a standstill. Your body will adjust and you will suddenly find your weight stabilizing. This has been my experience with running, but not with Phentermine. That's not to say that your body won't ever get use to the Phentermine as well. It's just that it will take longer than two weeks. I feel that the calorie-burning phenomenon is perhaps a more valuable quality than the appetite suppression. In either case, the calorie burning effect generally lasts longer than the appetite suppression. But the fact remains that eventually Phentermine wears off in its effectiveness. Your body will adjust to its effects just like it does to the jogging. It's just too hard to fight your breeding. It's also another reason to limit your time on Phentermine to 6 months.

This allows your body to regain some of the sensitivity to the Phentermine.

One bad thing about the low-carbohydrate diet is that it is very constipating. Poop is made of the things in our diet that do not get digested. A key ingredient is fiber, which is not digested. Doctors tell us to eat plenty of fiber containing foods, so that you can have a good BM every day without lots of straining. Now I've just told you to stop eating the foods that contain the most fiber, bread and cereal. So you are left with very little to move your bowels with. That's why I really push the second drug called Orlistat. When I started this book, it was listed as Xenical, which is available only by prescription. But by the time I finish this book, it will also be known as the over-the-counter version called Alli™. Orlistat works by blocking the digestion of fat. This means that you will be pooping fat instead of fiber. There are advantages and disadvantages to this fact.

When you are eating a low-carbohydrate diet, that generally implies that you will be eating more fat. That means that the Orlistat(Alli™) can further reduce your calories by taking the fat out of your diet. It's thought to eliminate 35% of fat from the diet. The undigested fat works it way through the bowels to be eliminated through defecation. The fat is actually a far better laxative than fiber. Fat is slippery and acts as a lubricant. It is also less solid, and therefore less bulky. This means that the fat works its way through the bowel much faster than the fiber. That is why two of the most widely used laxatives are oils, mineral oil and castor oil. Eliminating carb from your diet will actually make you look thinner, because fiber has a longer transit time than undigested fat. With Orlistat (Alli™), the fat you eat today should be gone tomorrow. With Raisin Bran, the fiber you eat today may take 48-72 hours to effect its escape. You may have a bowel movement every day by eating a bowl of Raisin Bran, but you can expect to poop today what you ate 2 or 3 days ago. All of that fiber takes up space. I know this first hand. Every now and then I used to eat a very large bowl of Raisin Bran, because I still like bran cereals. But I am doing it less and less, because I have come to expect to go two days without a BM while I wait for the very slow fiber to work its way through my bowel. It's like a slow moving semi on a country two-lane highway with a trail of fast moving cars that can't pass. In fact, the last time I ate a bowl of Raisin Bran I became nauseated, because it felt like I had a bowel obstruction. I didn't eat anything for the entire next day because of the nausea and bellyache. The fact is fiber takes up a lot of space. So, if you eat a high fiber diet, you are literally full of crap. They say that Elvis Presley had between 40 and 60 pounds of stool in his colon. His problem wasn't due to excessive fiber; it was a combination fast food and drugs that backed up his colon. I point out Elvis' problem simply to illustrate that the bowels can hold a lot of crap that can weigh you down. Nonetheless, it is thought that the average person will have 5 to 10 pounds of stool waiting in the colon. I maintain that a low carbohydrate diet with consistent use of Orlistat(Alli™) greatly reduces that figure, and that helps you look thinner quickly.

If you go to websites related to Orlistat(www.myalli.com), they do not encourage you to take Orlistat with the idea that you are going to eat a lot of fat. They actually think that your bowel is going to teach you a lesson if you eat a lot of fat, because they feel that the profuse defecation that ensues after a high-fat meal will discourage you from doing it again. My answer to that is 'go ahead, make my day!' I take it the to the other extreme. If I'm pooping, I'm losing! Orlistat isn't worth a crap, unless you're crapping. There is no point in taking Orlistat if choose to stay with a low-fat diet. The manufacturer still maintains the orthodox teaching that you should lose weight by general calorie reduction with the addition of Orlistat. They even tell you to eat lean and cut fat. But that is suboptimal use of a great product. By eliminating carbohydrates and then adding Orlistat, you are placing yourself on a high protein diet. This is what body-builders do to get the fat off while maintaining their muscle. So again I am a heretic in that I am pushing Orlistat with a high-fat diet. However, you can't argue with success, and I am convinced that I am much thinner in appearance, because I am not full of crap. So, rather than use excessive BM's as a sign that I am eating too much fat, I prefer to use constipation as a sign that I am eating too much carbohydrate.

To summarize my first line plan, I use Phentermine to suppress the appetite and to keep your body burning calories. In addition to the Phentermine I add in the Alli^{TM}, which is to be taken sometime between an hour before you eat to an hour afterward. My recipe for success is to start the day off with a Phentermine, skip breakfast, and then take the Alli^{TM}, two pills twice a day with meals. That's right I'm limiting you to two meals a day. Furthermore, I am committing further heresy by telling you to skip breakfast. Every health teacher I ever had has told me that breakfast is the most important meal of the day, because it gets your day started right. But what is breakfast? It is 'break' 'fast'; it means that you are breaking your fast. It is an excellent way to reverse the process whereby your body burns fat, because you start to bring calories into your body, often in the form of carbohydrates. If you bypass breakfast, you can gain another 5 to 7 hours of fat burning. Take the Phentermine and your hunger dissipates. I have tried eating breakfast and skipping lunch, but I have found that eating breakfast does nothing to diminish my desire for food at midday. I also find that many of my patients are relieved to be told by someone in my position that it's okay to skip breakfast. Years of guilt vanish with that instruction. Now, if you really want to eat 3 meals a day, you can, but it means that you will need 90 Xenical instead of 60 per month or 180 Alli™ instead of 120 per month, which brings me to the side effects section of this chapter.

We'll start with Phentermine. Most people love being on Phentermine. It generates a comfortable feeling of euphoria, not to the point that you're stoned and seeing angels in clouds while listening to Grateful Dead tunes. It's just a good feeling that leaves you feeling peppy and confident that you can handle anything that comes your way, especially your addiction to carbohydrates. People love the energy, which can also create productivity. But not everyone likes it. People who are prone to severe anxiety may find themselves terribly cranky. Some feel headaches. Others may feel heart palpitations. Phentermine can potentiate pain. I experienced this firsthand when I had a kidney stone in 2006. They were unable to knock me out despite massive doses of Demerol, Morphine, and Stadol.

In fact, after receiving these massive doses, I was still coherently telling my nurse(the one who works for me, not the one giving me the injections) when to reschedule my patients for surgery. More amazing was the fact that I had been up since 3 AM after delivering a baby. I even developed a peculiar heart rhythm called bigeminy, which really had my anesthesiologist worried. But I survived, and by the following Monday when I returned for my final treatment, I had no heart palpitations, because I was in virtually no pain. Others will describe difficulty with sleep, but I sleep incredibly well on Phentermine. I may sleep less, but I when I do sleep, its thoroughly deep and restful, the best sleep I have ever had. I believe that the increased metabolism wears you out, so that when you finally do get tired, you are so drained that sleep is restful. However, once it's time to get going, I take a Phentermine and off to work I go without nary a thought on sleep. As an Obstetrician, I am often called in the middle of the night. I have no problem going back to sleep if I'm tired. However, if I get called at 3AM to do a delivery, as I was when I had my kidney stone, I will often just stay up if the preceding nights have been restful ones. I find that I can tolerate minimal sleep for several nights in a row, but if I haven't been sleeping I find that I will make up for it on the subsequent night with a restful 9 or 10 hours of sleep. But I will still have a productive day in the office or wherever my duties take me until I reach bedtime. I can even take a nap on Phentermine if I'm tired. Personally, I love the way I sleep on Phentermine. But some will not like it. I also remind people that they don't need to sleep 8 hours per night. These are the people who seem most affected, because they still expect to go to bed every night at nine. Again, if you don't feel sleepy, stay up, read a book surf the internet, play a video game, exercise, spend some quality time with your significant other after the kids are in bed, or write a book like I'm doing. Even if you hardly slept 2 or 3 hours, your morning dose of Phentermine will keep you fully awake the next day. Nonetheless, I have seen some people cut the pills in half to reduce the dose if they feel over stimulated. However, I advise my patients that the body will build up a fairly fast tolerance to the stimulant attributes of the pills if they can just hang on 2 to 4 weeks. Cutting the pills in half will also reduce the benefits too. Unfortunately, there are some who cannot complete the program with the Phentermine due to feeling jittery. Some also complain of headaches, excessive insomnia, and irritability. The good news is that all adverse effects I have observed were reversed by simply stopping the medicine. Still, I rarely hear of someone who wants off of this effective and inexpensive medication.

Now for the side effects with Orlistat(Alli™). It has to do mostly with the defecation. Since I put patients on low carbohydrate diets, I expect them to poop more if they take Alli™. This is desirable with some such as myself, but it creates much anxiety in others. I often hear patients express these concerns, saying they know of someone who had an accident because of the grease in their stool. I am sure these things can happen. My key word of advice for those with such concerns is to avoid passing gas in public. Once you're on Alli™ (Orlistat), it becomes unsafe to assume that all that comes out is air. It is not unusual for the air to be intermingled with grease. The simple solution that I employ is to reserve all such activities for the toilet, because you never know what will come out when you let it rip. This is not all bad. Passing gas is a bodily function that is often shared between couples much to the disdain of the non-offending partner/victim. As I quickly realized that passing gas was no longer a safe way to antagonize my wife, I was able to reduce the discord between she and I in our quiet moments together. Not to worry, however, I am sure that I found other ways to antagonize her as she is now my ex-wife, but at least she could no longer call me a flatulent oaf, because I reserved that activity strictly for the privy. I have also found that reducing public flatulence makes your friends like you better too. Thus I have had no embarrassing moments on Alli™ or Xenical. Nonetheless, I would be remiss if I didn't inform you that some simply don't tolerate the cramps and bloating that may come with use of Orlistat. I have been asked about how it may affect someone with irritable bowel. I believe in some cases it may stabilize it by giving you some consistency with your BM's. It does not necessarily give you diarrhea. In fact, I was on another medication that gave me profuse watery diarrhea to the point that I was going as often as 7 times in an evening. The added bulk that I got by blocking the digestion of fat greatly reduced the amount of diarrhea I was having. Furthermore, I was able to give up this offending, diarrhea inducing, diabetes medication by losing the weight I needed to lose, which has made my life much better.

I think the biggest thing that has hindered my patients from taking Orlistat has been associated with the cost. As I am writing, the cost of Xenical has risen to over $2.00

per pill. The over the counter version, Alli™, is as little as $60 for 120 pills, but it is half the strength of the Xenical version of Orlistat, so you need to take 2 pills at a time for maximum benefit. The Phentermine has been around much longer than Orlistat, so it can be purchased as a generic pill. But there is no generic for Orlistat. So, the Phentermine costs between 10-30 dollars per month, while the Alli™ is costing about $60-$80 locally.

I will also add a little bit about what we call contraindications. These are reasons why I would decline to offer these medications to patients. Alli™ has very few direct contraindications. They generally pertain to pregnancy and breast-feeding, which applies to all diet pills, because it's generally considered bad to restrict a diet in these ladies. I avoid offering Phentermine to anyone with active heart disease, such as any history of heart attacks, angina, or valvular heart disease. I am less concerned about mitral valve prolapse, because I have yet to be convinced that there is any real significance to that condition in the absence of irregular heartbeats requiring medication. Certain pulmonary(lung) diseases will also keep me from prescribing the medicine. I also avoid prescribing the Phentermine to people who require sedatives like Benzodiazepines that include Valium and Xanax, because stimulants exacerbate anxiety. Having said that, I will still prescribe it to people who suffer from depression, especially if they are depressed about their weight. I also offer it to diabetics and hypertensive individuals. Losing weight can often cure or improve each of these two conditions. In fact, I believe that Phentermine is an effective way to lower blood sugar, and I have successfully been able to take type 2 diabetics off of insulin with the assistance of Phentermine.

There are other medications currently available that I use, but they are either adjuncts or medications that I use when a patient has completed their 6 months on Phentermine. They are far more expensive than Phentermine, and they don't provide as profound a response. The most common one that I use is Meridia. Meridia is the brand name of Sibutramine. This is a pure appetite suppressant. I have found that you need to take it for several days before the profound appetite suppression hits. But that's all it does. It causes you to eat less, but it does nothing to rev up your metabolism, which means that while you reduce your eating, your body has the ability to reduce it's caloric requirement so as to block your weight reduction efforts. Thus while you eat less you also burn less. Weight loss occurs but at a much slower rate. I have used Meridia with my Phen/Alli™ treatment in order to reduce my hunger at night. Then I prescribe it for people to hold back their appetite when they come off of Phentermine. Its major downside is the cost. The namebrand version of Meridia is over $100-$130 per month. If cost wasn't a factor, I would actually put everyone on it with the Phen/Alli™. Then I could call it Phen/Mer/Alli™. This is what I have done during my 4th time through the program. But it would cost most over $180-$200 per month to use all three medications. I do have a few patients who are on the triple therapy. It seems the appetite suppressant effects of the Phentermine wanes with time, but I find that the Meridia induced appetite suppressant improves with time. The Phentermine is still important to rev up the metabolism, so I find that these three agents combine nicely for the most profound weight-loss protocol that doesn't involve surgery. The other good thing about Meridia is that there is no limit to how long one can be on the therapy. At least there is no evidence I have found that prolonged use can cause problems as in Phentermine. With Meridia I tend to eat a filling lunch which is still low-carb, and I often find that my hunger never returns for the entire day all the way til bedtime.

There is another medication I also use during the 'off-season'. By 'off-season' I refer to that period of time where my patients cannot take the Phentermine for 6 months out of the year. In addition to the Meridia and the Alli™ I also offer Strattera. Strattera is not FDA approved for the treatment of obesity. Instead it is approved for the treatment of ADD(Attention Deficit Disorder). It is not classified as a stimulant and therefore it is not a controlled substance. This means that its use is not as closely regulated for 'off-label' use as are controlled substances. A lot people have the misconception that drugs can only be used for their FDA approved indications. However, we quite often use medications for treatments that have never been directly approved by the FDA, nor recommended by the manufacturer. This is never more true than in my medical specialty of Obstetrics, where every single drug I have ever used to treat premature labor has never been approved for the treatment of premature labor. In fact, one drug which I use with regularity for the induction of labor, Cytotec, has had a specific recommendation against its use as a labor induction agent issued by the drug company that manufactures it. Nonetheless, its effectiveness as an induction agent has been supported by the American College Obstetrics and Gynecology. Many companies simply choose not to seek out certain indications due to cost and liability factors. Strattera has the known side effect of weightloss in those that take it. I find it to be well tolerated and safe. I take it at the time of my first meal of the day. It upsets my stomach if I don't eat soon after taking it. I believe it works by revving up the metabolism and it may help lower appetite as well as the Meridia. Not everyone can afford to take this combination of medications as each one, the Meridia and the Strattera, can be up to $150 per month, and the results are nowhere near as good as the use of Phentermine by itself. But I am hoping to avoid what I call the round trip by employing these medications during that 6-month period where Phentermine must be given up. By 'round-trip' I mean gaining back all of the weight that was lost during the 6 months while on Phentermine. One bit of good news is that many insurances will contribute to the cost of Strattera. I only paid $35 with my insurance.

So, my goal is to get the most out of program at the very beginning where the Phentermine is most profoundly effective. Those first 3 months are often where the most weight is lost. Thus, this is the time when patients must use this opportunity to develop their discipline, learn to eat less carbohydrates, break their addictions to the foods that promote getting fat, so that they don't just gain it back when they come off of the Phentermine. Those that fail to enter the program with the idea that they are going to make lifelong changes will simply return to their preprogram weights within a few short months. The medications are to engineer an entire lifestyle change that will allow someone to maintain a leaner body for the remainder of their life. Some of these changes may be difficult to maintain, which is why I have a combination of medications for the entire year, and I program that can be followed for the rest of one's life if that is what it takes.

There are many other medications for the treatment of obesity in development as this chapter is being written. There are also several medications available for treatment of other conditions that I have used or are available to assist in the treatment of obesity. But none of these already available medications have been able to improve on the effectiveness and cost of the above combinations. This is especially true of Phentermine, which can be purchased for as little as $10 at a neighborhood pharmacy. Still, I expect this area of pharmaceutical development to be one of the most significant areas of development in the next decade.

Some feel that use of medicine to treat obesity is a failure of will-power. I have tried to show that it is our physiology to eat when food is plentiful, so as to deposit fat on our bodies in order to prepare for impending periods of starvation that used to occur with regularity. Our physiology has simply failed to change with the times. For those who feel that we should be able to maintain our weights naturally, through disciplined eating, I argue that you are taking a rather narrow view of the issue. There was a natural discipline that maintained human weight during the last millennium. It was called starvation and malnutrition. Without mimicking the conditions of NAZI concentration camps, it is very hard for most of us to maintain slim figures in our society. I find it ironic that these same champions of natural weight control techniques are also proponents of birth control, which is entirely unnatural as well. No one seems to be critical of using birth control pills or sterilization, except for the Pope. The fact remains that if we took the same view toward family planning, we would find that most women would have 10-15 pregnancies during their reproductive years. So, I contend that if it is appropriate to use medicine and surgery to control the size of families, then why not use medication, and if necessary, surgery to control our abdominal girth?

Another issue I find is that people try to cut corners. There are two critical mistakes that I see. First, people are trying to skip out on the Alli™. Second, people don't come back every month for refills. When it was Xenical, I understood patients' aversion, because it was nearly $100 more per prescription. Now that Alli™ is cheaper, expense is less of an issue. I concede that if you are only looking to lose 20 pounds, you can accomplish that with just one medication, the cheap and efficacious Phentermine. But the people who need to lose more than 30 pounds really need the added benefits. Alli™ is a waistline shrinker, because it empties the bowels. I had a couple start the program who both weighed around 300 pounds. The man decided he didn't want to use Alli™ and the woman did. He still lost weight with a ten pound reduction, but she lost 22. Every woman resents men for their ability to lose weight in greater quantities, yet here this woman not only lost more weight in the first month, she doubled him. Needless to say, Alli™ is going to get you more out of this program, but I have to do more persuading with that one due to the increased cost and fear of excessive pooping. I remember one girl at a seminar asked me, "Is it true it gives you nasty poops?"

I replied, "I've never seen a poop that wasn't nasty."

Of course, I'm told there are some people who think their poops don't stink, but I think that was a metaphor for arrogance. The fact remains that Alli™ is the best way to avoid having to choose between high-carb fiber and constipation.

Skipping months or weeks poses a different problem. As soon as you come off the Phentermine, especially if it's only been one or two months, your body rebounds much harder, because of all the starvation reflexes. I've seen people do two or three months and return 12 months later only to weigh more than when they started. Or they skip a month and come in weighing only 2 pounds less than their last visit. That probably means that they lost a good amount of weight and regained 90% of it back. I explain that they are paying good money to lose weight that they already paid money to lose. I tell people not to do this program until they can devote 6 straight months to it, because you can't lose over 30 pounds without devotion.

Again, if you are one of those people who want to lose less than 20 pounds you may be done with the program within a few months. You have more flexibility. In fact, I recommend hitting it hard for 2 or 3 months if you're one of those '20 or unders' like my wife. Then I recommend keeping some Phentermine on hand to take as needed at the first sign of rebounding back up. My wife went from 170 to about 148 in two months. She went from a size 12 to a size 8 in two months and had to stop, because she was losing too much weight. Now she just takes them after the holidays or when she has a bad week of overindulgence.

The important thing to emphasize is that these medications aren't like antibiotics, which one must merely take to be cured of their ailment. You have to do your part. Alter your eating, come consistently for your refills, and use both medications for maximum effect. If you do that, there can only be success.

6

Misleading Labeling

Are you still confused? Not sure what has excessive carbohydrates? Here is an opportunity to get a primer on how to read the ingredients on the container of most food and drink. Every processed food, i.e. anything that is packaged for mass production will provide a list of ingredients along with other nutritional information. Anyone who is on a diet should make a point of inspecting these labels in order to avoid mistakes in food selection. Information that is usually included will be the number of calories, the number of servings, the size of the serving, the breakdown of carbs, fats, and proteins. Many times the carbs will be broken down into sugars versus other carbs. The FDA requires this kind of product labeling. Fresh fruit, vegetables, and meats will not have this kind of information. However, if you use my simple guideline, you shouldn't need a label. Plant products get their calories from carbohydrates and meats get their calories from fat and protein. For the purpose of this chapter though, we will concern ourselves with processed foods.

Keep in mind that the manufacturers of these foods are well aware that most Americans struggle with their weight, and therefore, they will do everything they can to convince you that you support your weight loss efforts by consuming their product. In order to see through their marketing ploys, it is imperative that you learn to turn the box over to the side or back so that you can get the details on just what is contained in a box or serving of this product. The details on the back are required by law and must be factual and there is no room for deception. What appears on the front of the container is open to interpretation. Makers of various products can assert all sorts of claims, which are vague or subjective. That's where you see phrases like 'less carbs', 'low fat', 'healthy', 'light' and 'diet'. These are comparative terms and you have no idea what they are comparing themselves to. Thus, there is no way to disprove the claims, which leads to apparently contradictory terminology in food description like low-carb cookies even though there is no way to make a low carb cookies or bread. Sure, they have less carbs than the average slice, but they still get all of their calories from carbohydrate. So, let's work through some of the claims that we see on the package.

One of my favorite misleading labels is "no sugar added." In actuality, there is nothing deceptive at all about this labeling. Indeed the producers of these products don't add sugar, but they are relying on you to misconstrue the meaning to imply sugar free. So, when you see this form of labeling, I generally recommend that you discard this type of product. This usually implies that the product has enough sugar in it already so that no more sugar is required. It is impossible to make these products sugar free because they are derived from high sugar products. This is a common labeling with tart, fruity things like jellies, juices, and dried fruit. These products are all sugar. They may not have table sugar added, but they are still usually 100% carbohydrate. Don't get duped into partaking in these treats. My feeling is that if I'm going to have something like that, I might as well get the normal stuff, because if I'm going to cheat I might as well get the most out of it.

Having made a distinction between "no sugar added" and "sugar free," I still need to warn you that "sugar free" doesn't always mean no carbohydrates. Sugar is technically sucrose, better known as table sugar, but it's not the only sugar out there. Remember, all carbohydrates are sugars. Complex carbohydrates are chains of individual sugar molecules called monosaccharides. These molecules are known as glucose and fructose. Sucrose is a disaccharide which has two sugar molecules consisting of one glucose and one fructose molecule. Hence, eliminating sucrose still leaves all manner of simple and complex carbs available to place in the product while still declaring itself "sugar free". I just went online to see some the available products that fit this description. On a website that is devoted to 'sugar free' products I found a 'sugar free' pancake mix. While there is no sucrose, there are 26 grams of other carbohydrates per serving. I can imagine many of my patients consuming mass quantities of this product in good conscience only to find out that they were inadvertently carb loading. That's why it's so important to read the labels.

If the sugar serves as the sole source of calories, and we take all of the sugar out of it and replace it with an artificial sweetener that has no calories then we are onto something. That's the case with many drinks like Diet Coke, Crystal Lite, and sugar free sweet teas. While we are on the topic of 'sugar free', let's talk about the sugar alcohols. These are indeed carbohydrates and they taste sweet, but your body cannot burn these sugars for energy as well as sugar. They do not raise your blood sugar or effect your insulin levels. However, they do have calories, but it is still controversial as to whether they constitute carbohydrate calories or another classification of unto themselves. Gram for gram, sugar alcohols have between 25% and 75% of the calories found in sucrose. These sugar alcohols are often used in gums and candies. Sorbitol and mannitol are examples of these. The other thing to be aware of is the fact these agents are not well absorbed into the blood stream so they tend to work their way through the colon, where bacteria can also use them for energy. The bacteria convert the sugar alcohols to energy and gas, which can lead to cramping, bloating, and flatulence. In as much as I recommend Orlistat for my patients, which prohibits the public passing of gas, the use of excessive sugar alcohols can prove discomforting. So, be careful not to overdo it with the sugar alcohols. I have paid the price on more than one occasion by consuming excessive sugar-free chocolate. Let's just say that I didn't get much sleep the following night.

Now for the true no-calorie artificial sweeteners. Nutra-sweet is the branded version of Aspartame. Aspartame revolutionized the diet drink industry. Before Aspartame, we were stuck with Saccharine, also know as Sweet-n-Low. It was found in Tab, the only diet soda around when I was a kid. Then in 1981 Aspartame was approved for use in diet drinks and other products. That's when I started drinking diet sodas. Aspartame is still the most widely used sugar substitute in America, but I still like to sweeten ice tea with Saccharine. You can tell the two brands apart by their familiar packets, blue for Aspartame and pink for Saccharine. Now there's also a yellow packet and that's Splenda, the branded version of the chemical sweetener known as Sucralose. Through a chemical process the makers of Splenda start with sucrose and add chlorine atoms to the sugar molecule to render the sugar unusable by the body, but it retains its sweetness. Not only does it retain its sweetness it is reportedly 600 times sweeter than sugar. Splenda has thoroughly challenged Nutra-Sweet for artificial sweetener supremacy. In fact, the makers of Nutra-Sweet recently sued the makers of Splenda. Don't ask me why. It's of no consequence to this book, having more to do with marketing issues. What is of consequence are the allegations of rampant toxicity among the artificial sweeteners, especially Aspartame. Aspartame has been around much longer than Splenda, but I am starting to see that the conspiracy theorists are starting their assaults on Splenda as well. The fact remains, despite these allegations, that thorough FDA approved studies have failed to confirm or verify a single allegation against either of these two sweeteners. These claims are perpetuated by groups and individuals in search of a cause for whatever malady is affecting them. When you encounter these claims, just remember it's easy to claim anything. Proving an allegation is a whole other proposition. None of these claims have arisen out of scientific journals or highly scrutinized data. Someone can claim anything from a website, blog or even a book that they happen to be writing but that doesn't mean it's true. I prefer to go with the mainstream scientific data at this point. Having said that, I recognize that I am an author writing a book with sensational claims that haven't been published elsewhere. But my work represents a synthesis of data form various sources that have evidence to support them individually. I am offering two FDA approved medications, which require data for approval, and there is data to support the low-carb diet as the most effective diet in America. So now I am coming out in support of using Aspartame and Splenda in place of Sucrose, yet another recommendation based on scientifically derived facts. I don't have a preference between the two in terms safety and caloric content, though I personally prefer Aspartame, but that's a personal choice. Just bear in mind as always, sugar free does not guarantee you carbohydrate free.

So when you look at the back of the box under carbohydrates. You will see it subdivided into sugars and fibers. Sugars are generally calories from simple carbs, usually sucrose. So subtracting the sugar grams from the total grams will tell you the amount of complex carbs. Fibers are considered complex carbs. I have a few examples taken from my own cupboard. Before you start calling me a hypocrite for my high-carb indulgences, keep in mind that these were purchased by my wife for her own kids. This may shed some light on why there is a major obesity problem in this country. Carb addictions start early. Let's start with generic oatmeal. It has 26 grams of total carbohydrate. There is 0 sugar 4 grams of fiber. This makes oatmeal carbs 100% complex carbs. Let's compare that to All-Bran crackers by Kellogg's. Total carbs are 19, sugars 3, fiber 5, meaning 16 out of 19 carbs are complex. Remember complex carbs take longer to burn, because they have to be broken down to individual carb molecules. Next, let's look at a sugary cereal—something I grew up on like Apple Jacks. Total carbs are 30. 16 are sugars and there's one gram of fiber. So how many complex carb grams? 14. Let's see what my stepkids are snacking on that's not a 'sweet'. We have Stax by Lays with Sunflower Oil giving 0 grams of trans fats. Total carbs are 16 per serving, 0 sugar carbs and 1 fiber carb. But what is the serving size? 13 chips. When was the last time you ate 13 chips only? So, there are 100% complex carbs in this product. They're trying to make you feel good about yourself because you are eating no trans fats. The presence or absence of trans fats is irrelevant to our diet, because when you go low carb, any fat is okay. It's the carbs that go with them that get you. So don't be lured by claims that are irrelevant to the prescribed low carbohydrate diet.

Another pitfall is the serving size of a product. A common mistake is to assume that the entire box or package represents one serving. It's an expected assumption that most people like us have a strong appetite and can eat the entire container in one sitting. However, many times the manufacturer of this product will divide it into multiple servings. It's listed right there on the box so it's not technically deceptive. They are counting on you to deceive yourself. The classic one is the 20-oz soda. It will list the calories as 100 per serving. 100 calories do not seem like all that much, but they define their servings as 8 ounces not 20. They also list servings per container as 2 and ½. So in actuality a 20-ounce soda with sugar has 250 calories. So pay attention to servings per container and serving size when considering choosing a product. The manufacturers are counting on you to overlook such details. Just look at the above Stax label. 13 chips is a serving. I for one am more than capable of eating the entire container in one sitting. That's 6 servings at 900 calories and 96 grams of complex carbs.

While we are here let's talk about some other concepts that are out there. For example, many websites are touting the term 'net' carbs. By this accounting of carbs people are claiming that you can subtract certain carbs from the total carbs like fiber carbs. They claim that these carbs do not count because you do not digest them for calories, therefore they have no effect on blood sugar. While this is true, I am a firm opponent of high fiber diets when Orlistat(Alli^{TM}) is being used. This is not because of the caloric and glycemic issues, rather, this is due to the long transit time through the gut, which contributes to your abdominal girth just as much as fat does. So, I urge you not to ignore these carbs. I am not of the opinion that there are good carbs, but I believe that all complex carbs are to be avoided. If you must have carbs I believe that simple carbs are the best, because they are most rapidly consumed and they are absorbed ready to burn. There are many Atkin's labeled products that are fiber rich that I do not advocate.

Patients are constantly asking me about what's allowed. The fact is you shouldn't have to ask, because I get my answers the same place you can—the sides of packages. But before I close this chapter I will give you some ingredient advice on things that you don't often have an opportunity to evaluate because they don't come in packages. Soybeans are often construed to be pure protein they are not. They are like most beans. Here is one package that breaks down a serving of soy nuts. They have 8 grams of fat, 13 grams of protein and a total of 8 grams of carbs, 6 of which are complex. You can't eat these or any other nuts or beans under the assumption that you are enjoying a low carb treat. Let's look at fruits. I have been an advocate of avocado consumption, which is the main ingredient of Guacamole since I undertook this diet. But the fact remains, I haven't actually looked up the carb/nutrient content of various fruits and vegetable until now. So, I have to see how I've done. Let's see how various fruits break down per 100 grams of each product. Avocado has 190 total calories, 5.3 grams of carbs, 1.9 grams of protein, and 19.5 grams of fat. 3.4 grams of the avocado is in the form of fiber. An apple has 47 calories, 13.6 total carbs, 0.4 grams of protein, and 0.1 grams of fat. A banana has 95 calories, 24.3 grams of carb, 1.2 grams of protein, and 0.3 grams of fat. Melon has 24 calories, 6.2 grams of carb, 0.6 grams of protein, and 0.1 grams of fat. While there are more calories per 100 grams of avocado than any other fruit, only 20% of avocado carbs come from carb. Bananas represent the worst source of fruit carbs with 24.3 grams of carbs. They are virtually 100% complex carbs with very little fiber. While I am not a huge advocate of ignoring fiber calories, they are better than other complex carbs. The carbs in avocado are 60% fiber. The one thing that fiber will not do is keep your from burning fat. Eat a banana and you won't burn fat for quite some time, because they are complex carbs that disrupt the fat burning process. I am amazed at how many women come to me thinking they are doing something healthy by eating bananas. Personally, I love bananas, but they are one of the worst cheats on my diet. The other good thing about the avocado is that it is a better source of potassium than banana. By better I mean better for the diet, not necessarily richer in potassium than bananas. It's also interesting to note how little carb there is in melons. The problem I see with melons is at buffets. Most people eat so many pieces of precut melon without seeds that they end up eating a pound of the stuff, which turns it into a 25 gram carb treat as opposed to a 5.5 gram treat. So with regard to fruit, one a day won't destroy the diet, but don't make it the key ingredient of your meals, except for avocado. Eat nothing but avocado and take your Orlistat with it and your on your way.

7

Natural is Not Necessarily Better

So many people are wrapped up in the word 'natural'. They want natural hormones. They want natural childbirth. They want organic products. Bill Engvall even has a comedy bit about his wife's desire to only eat 'free range' chickens. Hence, I spend much of my time explaining why I don't believe in the natural approach to certain treatments. Don't get me wrong. Natural is better in certain circumstances. After all, our species has made it all these millenniums without many options other than natural. Thus, many will conclude that what was good for the hunter-gatherers should suffice for the 21st century. I just don't think natural works best in all circumstances. Leaving the sex of your baby to natural chance is a pretty good option, one which I applied for all three of my own kids, but there is technology that is claimed to help a person choose the sex of their offspring. While we're on the subject of procreation, I will add that when it comes to making babies, I without a doubt prefer natural methods as opposed to test tube babies. However, there are those where natural reproduction is not an option due to infertility. For such people I am glad that artificial techniques are available. So, I ask those who insist on natural techniques: What do you do when natural doesn't get it done?

My favorite argument against arbitrarily siding in favor of natural modes of survival is suggesting a trip to a cemetery that is over 60 years old. That's where you find the remains of those that were forced to live exclusively by the natural method. All we have to do is travel to the Harmony Cemetery in Pocahontas, Arkansas, which is located in the original 40 acre Burtman farm. Now it is a public cemetery. My grandmother is buried there. She was pregnant 14 times from the age of 17 to the age of 46. She had her kids between the years of 1928 and 1957. This time period encompassed the great depression years. They were poor farmers, but they did own the land they lived on. My grandmother had all but her last child at home. She was fortunate enough to survive all of her deliveries. Of the 14 pregnancies 13 produced live babies. She had one miscarriage. But she also had a surprise on her 3rd delivery. The midwife discovered a 2nd baby after delivering my Uncle Herald. She was unable to deliver that 2nd baby, which resulted in a stillbirth. Clearly, the ability to do an ultrasound would have saved that baby and given me an additional uncle, because the high-risk delivery could have been done in a hospital with an obstetrician trained in delivering twins or performing Cesarean Sections. Of the remaining 13 babies, 2 died in infancy and 2 others died under unusual circumstances. One allegedly received a home remedy containing Arsenic that may have killed her. The youngest died at the age of 2 when he drowned in the pond on the farm. My grandmother had entrusted his care to my teenage uncles who simply forgot to watch him. Naturally, no one was there to do CPR after they pulled him from the water, but that wouldn't have been natural to resuscitate a drowning toddler like that. Thus I never knew my Uncle Paul Allen who died 5 years before I was born.

Go to any cemetery near your home that goes back to the depression and you will see numerous gravesites with a woman's grave who was in her 20's and next to it a small child's grave. You may see that the child's birthday corresponds with the date that the mother died, and very likely the same day that the child also died. Just look at the ages of the adults in the graves. Take note that the further back you go, the younger the average age is. I remember asking my father during our visits to cemeteries how my great great grandfather could have had 3 wives without ever getting divorced. My father explained that his wives kept dying of natural causes. Then I asked how my great great grandfather could father a child at the age of 79. He explained that when a woman was widowed with children back then there was no welfare to fall back on. Thus a widow often depended on an elderly man to support them while they cared for him and satisfied his needs. Before the days of Viagra that may not have required much activity in the bedroom either. However, my Civil War Veteran great great grandfather still had some life left in him. Way to go Great Great Grandpa!

That child was born in 1926. We called him Uncle Charley. He was the most pleasant man I ever knew. But he was a child before there were polio vaccines, and he came down with the polio virus when he was about 11. He lost use of all but his left hand. Nonetheless, he managed to get married twice with a long hiatus between marriages in which he lived alone, cared for himself, and got around town in a powered wheelchair. He was great on the harmonica, but he even found a way to play a little slide guitar. Interestingly, he was one of the last people to draw a pension check from the Civil War, because dependents of Civil War Veterans were eligible to receive the benefits.

I know many of you may have found the above to be a mere exercise in bragging about my family or complaining about the poor health/judgment of my forbears. However, I want to point out that these outcomes are par for most rural Southern families. Then I hope you can already see that every misfortune detailed could have been avoided had the technology that's commonplace today been employed 60 or so years ago. With modern medicine all 13 of those children might have survived—even Paul Allen could have survived had CPR been utilized at the scene. My Uncle Charley would have received a polio vaccine preventing his lifetime of imprisonment in his wheelchair.

We can even take it one step further. Back then my grandmother was not unusual in having 14 pregnancies. Indeed that was typical back then, but now 14 kids would be worthy of Ripley's Believe It Or Not, because we have birth control. These days it's rare to see women have more than four babies. Many consider it irresponsible to have that many. Ironically, the natural approach would yield something more like my grandmother. The fact is we have used technology to create birth control pills or sterilization techniques to impair our natural fertility. Guess what that means. If you are on a birth control pill or have had your tubes tied, you are indeed abnormal either physiologically or anatomically, and that's not natural. But most of you are like, so what! But that's precisely my point—so what if it's not natural. Natural, i.e. having 14 babies by the time your 50, isn't always the best thing for you. Hence, we make ourselves abnormal, i.e. unnatural, in order to prevent the excessive child bearing that would otherwise be in store for us.

So, as a woman or as a man married to or dating a fertile woman, how would you feel if the doctor, when asked for birth control, advised you or your mate to simply have less sex? You'd probably change doctors. Yet I argue that is precisely what your doctor does when he or she refuses to offer you medication to help with weightloss.

The natural order of things for women especially is to get pregnant and have a baby about once every 15 months. These deliveries are painful and life-threatening to both mother and baby. After a 30-40 year reproductive lifespan, a woman can celebrate the end to child bearing with menopause, which while freeing a woman of her menstrual cycles (yet another natural physiologic pain in the backside), still results in osteoporosis, accelerated aging, diminished sexual response, and the loss of the one hormone that maintains her femininity. Add to that the natural tendency to gain weight with each pregnancy, the physiologic responses to appetizing sensations, and the natural tendency to gain weight when there is never a naturally imposed scarcity of food, and natural just ain't all it's cracked up to be.

It's indeed ironic that we seem to intervene for every aspect of a woman's natural though somewhat adverse life events. We offer birth control pills to control the size of the family, analgesia to make having a baby more comfortable, prenatal care and other interventions like ultrasounds, forceps, and C/sections in order to prevent losses of mothers and babies, surgeries along with other treatments for heavy, painful periods, and finally we can completely reverse menopause by giving back the hormones that are naturally eliminated. However, go ask your primary physician for some diet pills, and he tells you that you need to eat less and exercise more. I hate to say it, but physicians are late to adapt to the natural consequences of improved technology and resources. In the United States that means obesity, which is the natural result of plentiful food among people who are especially well adapted to survive starvation. To me, providing diet pills is no different than providing birth control pills to reproductive age females. Both interventions render a woman abnormal, unnatural as it were, but the results are most desirable—limited offspring and limited waistlines. Both interventions carry certain risks, but the benefits outweigh the risks for most. There are those who should not be on diet pills, just as there are those who aren't good candidates for birth control pills. That's why you need to see a doctor for either type of pill. But to say that we should limit diet pills to the most extreme cases is like saying we should limit birth control pills to nymphomaniacs. The fact is I don't see why we shouldn't use these diet medications to prevent morbid obesity. Waiting until a person reaches a certain critical mass is like refusing to give a woman birth control pills until her family reaches a certain size. We know that women who do nothing to curtail their breeding will have upwards of ten babies by the time she is 50. Likewise we know that Americans become obese simply by eating according to the normal federal guidelines mandating a balanced diet comprised of the portions from all 4 food groups. Why prevent one natural consequence of normal human behavior with medication and refuse to prevent another. Obesity has numerous adverse consequences. Diabetes, heart disease, arthritis, stroke, and secondary problems like kidney failure are all consequences of obesity. The aforementioned diseases account for 50% of all deaths annually in the USA. Infections account for an additional 6% of all deaths. Many of these infections are actually a coup de grace to other chronic disease processes that leave patients vulnerable to the infections which directly kill them. So these may be an indirect consequence of the other obesity related diseases. Yet many physicians still play the improve your diet and exercise card, claiming that natural trumps intervention this one time. The only way we will naturally defeat obesity is if an asteroid strikes earth and creates havoc that destroys our food supply, technology, and economic stability. Then the obese will survive through natural selection while the skinny aerobics instructors die of starvation, because their hyperactive metabolisms offer them no caloric reserves. Then we can go back to the good old days of starvation, death and disease that came with nature that offered no unnatural alternatives.

8

Living by the Method

More than four years have passed since I first embarked on this thing I refer to as the Burtman Method of Weight loss. I have gone from a peak weight of 245 to as low as 212 pounds. Now I reside consistently between 213 and 218, occasionally a little more sometimes a little less. This week I weighed even less at 213. As I have progressed further down the road, I have had lower peaks and I have stayed more consistently below the above range rather than over it. Actually, I don't weigh myself very often; instead, I follow my belt. I still wear the same belt I had when I weighed 245 as a reminder of the former breadth of my waistline. The marks from previous use are still evident in the holes where the buckle secured the leather. As a weight management clinician, I am for more sympathetic to the plight of those who crave certain delectable treats. After all, I am human first, physician second. I still admit that I have a carb addiction, and I further concede that I do give in to certain urges from time to time. This chapter deals with the day to day living within the framework of my plan. I will give you some ideas as to how I maintain myself on my good days, and how I selectively choose to cheat. I admit that there is a difference between the theoretical side and the realistic human approach that I live by. As you read this I also want you to be mindful of the fact that I was quite faithful to the plan when I was losing my 33 pounds.

Only then did I begin to drift, as I became satisfied with what I had accomplished. The same need for fidelity was not as requisite when I was merely trying to maintain the weightloss I had already accomplished. In order to lose weight, you have to be more strict, and the more you need to lose to reach your goals, the longer you must maintain that fidelity to the ideal plan. Once you see the results you desire, then there are ways to sin and pay less of a price in pounds.

My ideal day starts with no breakfast. I have had nothing to eat since the night before, so my body must depend on fat to maintain its metabolism. Eating breakfast would simply put an end to that process. In as much as I have always managed without breakfast, this required no adjustment on my part. I do start with a diet soda. That's just my preference. For you it may be coffee. Cream would be a fine additive, but no sugar. Non-caloric artificial sweeteners would be fine. I also take a phentermine if it's during my 6 months of the year that I am allowed to be on it. I will be fairly content with nary a thought of food until lunch time. Those that use the fact that they eat out a lot as an excuse for failing to maintain the program see little sympathy from me, because 80% of my meals are not prepared at home. I have managed to find low-carb entrées at every restaurant imaginable. Monday lunch will often consist of a chicken Cordon-bleu, a creamy chicken noodle soup as my side, and perhaps a salad with blue-cheese dressing to start. On Tuesday we often grab the Pizza Hut buffet. We eat no bread sticks or dessert pizza, and I try to stick to thin crust, avoiding the rim of pure crust, but I still eat the flat part of the crust at the center. I even get some extra sauce for dipping the pizza. If I'm on my own for lunch, I will get the Low-Carb Burger at Hardees, which is two patties with cheese wrapped in lettuce, and it's loaded with all of the fixins. There is a sub sandwich place in town. I like the chicken salad, but I noticed that you get more chicken salad if you order the big sandwich instead of just the chicken salad salad. So I simply order the footlong chicken salad sandwich, and eat the chicken salad off of the bread. I also like to get a boneless buffalo wing wrap and dip it in blue cheese or ranch dressing. If I'm going more formal, I like a big steak with a salad, perhaps a side of mushrooms. At Outback Steakhouse, they offer a side of shrimp or crablegs, which makes a great low-carb addition to your meal. I hope you are beginning to pick up on a theme here. What am I leaving off of the list? Potatoes! When my appetite goes down, I am more than satisfied without requiring a loaded baked potato or fries. Eating out is about the easiest way to maintain the low-carb diet.

Nonetheless, low-carb diets do require planning. For example, if you work somewhere that requires you to stay put for lunch, like a school or factory, you have to plan ahead, because snack machines are not known for the their low-carb selections. My suggestion is to pack your lunch in those cases. An easy thing to pack is canned tuna. In place of sandwiches you can pack wraps. Pork rinds are the best crunchy snack out there. Beef jerky has become a widespread treat because it is such a high protein snackfood, although it does tend to have sugar in it. Despite the presence of sugar, it is still a good adjunct to a home lunch because it's not very much sugar and it's all simple sugar. If you have access to a microwave, left over pizza and fried chicken are good for lunch.

Now that I mentioned fried chicken, lets talk about breaded things. People ask me, "Hey, isn't there carb in the breading?"

And they are absolutely correct; the breading is carbohydrate. However, I consider those carbs to be incidental carbs. The normal KFC diner tends to load up on biscuits, potatoes and gravy, corn on the cob, beans, and a whole host of other high carb sides. By sticking to just chicken, you eliminate 90% of the carbs available on the KFC menu. Remember, you developed your weight problem by indulging in all the other parts of the menu. It's not the breading that made you fat. It's everything else on the menu that you have now eliminated. I have also noticed that people who eat nothing but baked, skinless chicken with a salad, don't lose as much weight as my normal fried food consumers. I remind people that I think it's important to indulge in the things you like that you are allowed to have since I have forced you off of so many other things you do like. You don't get extra credit for torturing yourself.

Dinner can consist of a salad and steak. I just skip the big baked potato. But evening time is when I am most vulnerable to temptation. I think the biggest reason for that is the television. First, I enjoy eating while watching TV, so I am not eating out of a sense of hunger, but out of a sense of enjoyment. Secondly, the programming itself is going to drive your hunger reflexes crazy. Just seeing people eat will make you hungry. Then there are advertisements designed to arouse your appetite, and the next thing you know, you're making a stop at the refrigerator like a hypnotized zombie. This is when munching on pork skins or beef jerky can be employed. But like many of you, I can't do that every night. What I do is try to find myself other activities so that I'm not parked in front of the TV. Since my weightloss activities started, I have launched some new activities for myself to keep me away from my TV and available food. I have joined a rock band, and I have purchased a little old theater in my hometown of Columbus, Mississippi. This has given me many other activities to participate in to keep me out from the couch. But I understand that not everyone has the luxury or time to do such things.

For those who are still vulnerable to sinning against the program, I have devised a sort of hierarchy of sins. I'm sure we will all fall short of the diet plan that I propose. I am no exception. What I have found though are ways to get away with cheating by avoiding the very worst mistakes. But make no mistake about it, these are still sins.

First, I will go into what kind of foods cost you the most. Remember that carbohydrates come in two forms—complex and simple. Complex carbs are especially bad because they must first be broken down to simple carbs before your body can use them for energy. So, it takes your body much longer to use them up before your body once again has any need to burn fat. Contrast this to simple carbs, which are immediately available to be burned. This means that while your blood sugar levels spike up rapidly, they also are quickly burned up, especially if you've been starved of carbs all day. Before long you will go back to burning fat again. Thus, I advocate using sweets over starches if one must eat something that is off of the diet.

The worst things are things that are high in both fat and complex carbs. That would mean that potato chips would top the list of sins. Adding dip would make it even worse. Also included in that list would be chips of all kinds, including corn chips, tortilla chips, crackers, wheat thins, and cheesy chips of all kinds. Pork skins are the only crunchy chips out there that have zero carbs.

Next on my list of sins are the cakes and cookies. These are mostly complex carbs, but also have fat and loads of sugar added. We can include pancakes, waffles, French toast, and all breakfast confectioneries. Even if you see 'sugar free' on the label, there is enough complex carbs on board to destroy all of your dieting efforts for the day.

Many find it surprising to hear me say that chocolate is better than potato chips. I include ice cream in that category as well. I prefer that you eat these types of things because they are devoid of complex carbs. They are high in simple carbs. If you've been good all day on your ultra-low-carb diet, then your body will be soaking up and burning carbs like a dry sponge. This means that you will burn these carbs quickly. They won't hang around like the complex carbs found in pastries and chips. Complex carbs have to be converted to simple carbs before they can be burned, so you stop burning fat longer when you eat them. So if you must cheat, do so with sweet carbs, because you will get them out of your system sooner.

You can get away with cheating when you are in the maintenance mode, but it still must not become regular event in your life. While the primary medications are prescribed for 6 months, I do not look at this program as a 6-month program. You have to maintain as well as possible your carbohydrate reduction lest you make the round trip back to your starting weight. It's just like birth-control pills. No one takes them with the expectation that they will be on them for 6 months only, and then go back to having unprotected sex. But I do understand that your urges may get the better of you from time to time. The key is to make addition of carbs as rare a treat as possible instead of the mainstay of you diet.

I also advocate bingeing over nibbling. Every time you take in sugar, you stop burning fat. So, if you nibble on M&M's all day long you won't burn fat all day. You're better off eating the whole bag at one time later in the evening than having a few every 5 minutes all afternoon. If I have an irresistible urge to have doughnuts, I'll eat 5, but then I won't have anymore for a few months. I get it out of my system. They key is that I don't succumb to the urge on a daily basis. So, it is not as if you must say good bye to your favorite treats once and for all. You must simply relegate these things to rare treats instead of the staples of your every day menu.

Now nearly 5 years from my own attempt at the weightloss, I am wondering about another phenomenon. This past year has been the most stable year, in terms of weight, of my life. My weight has been below 218 for greater than one year. The way I wear the weight compares to how I looked when I weighed less than 200 pounds 20 years ago. I just have less hair on my head now. Recalling the body's tendency to want to maintain the status quo, I am wondering and hoping that my body will now recognize this new weight as my natural weight. I say this because it seems that my weight stays about the same now no matter what I eat. Granted, I don't eat any major potato servings, and I haven't had a bowl of cereal in 16 months, but I just don't see the fluctuations when I decide to eat a big pancake breakfast or feast on my mother-in-law's cooking. The point of this is that I am hoping that you will find your weightloss efforts easier to maintain as you maintain the weight you have lost. I expect that you will be most vulnerable to regaining your lost weight immediately after you lose it. This is when you must try your best to keep the pounds off. If you can hold off the rebounding weight gain for a matter of a few years, then you will find that you can get away with a few more treats as the years come and go. I know that I found myself bouncing back up all the way to 228 lbs after my first 6 months of Phentermine concluded, which is what prompted me to devise the Meridia and Strattera combination, because I was headed for the round trip back to 245. Using these two agents was critical to my maintenance. If you lose lots of weight only to gain it back on your 6 months off, I have to ask you what you are hoping to accomplish with your investment of time and money? So, the point is to do everything you can to keep the weight off once you lose it. It's as important as losing it in the first place. There are two key benefits to keeping the weight off as well. First, it creates a better opportunity to lose more weight when you come back for more Phentermine in another six months. Second, the longer you keep it off the easier it is to keep it off. You accomplish nothing if you lose as much as 100 pounds if gain it right back after you complete the first 6 months of the program.

9

OTHER WEIGHT LOSS PROGRAMS

My program is not the first weightloss program to succeed. In fact, I wouldn't go so far as to even call it my own program. My program is a combination of other established modalities. The medications were not developed by me, nor was the low carb diet. I doubt that I am the first person to ever devise this strategy either. I'm just trying to share my ideas, observations, and conclusions as a healthcare provider who has dealt extensively with weightloss issues both personally and professionally. It was never my ambition to become some expert on weightloss. It just worked out that way. This book is a byproduct of our success. Having said that, I am aware that there are other programs that have achieved some success in helping people lose weight. Even though I am writing a book touting 'my approach' to weightloss, I am not going to claim to be the only way to get there. The thing I need to emphasize is that if you want to lose weight you have to do something, and it usually has to be fairly radical to alter the balance in your body's metabolism. The medicine is there help you make the changes, but I am aware that there are many changes that may be made that may help you lose weight if the low carb approach does not work for you or is intolerable to you. There also alternatives to using medications as well.

First, let me discuss one weightloss program that is virtually assured to help you lose more pounds than my own program. It may surprise you that I would tout another approach as a way to lose more weight. *Why don't you write a book about that then?* I know you're asking yourself that one. Let me explain. It's because I think it's overkill for most patients. I also cannot offer this service to my patients, because I am not qualified to offer this kind of treatment. I am referring to gastric surgery.

Gastric surgery has made several advances recently with the development of the 'Lap Band' procedure. The idea is to shrink the stomach surgically. With the Lap Band, there is an external compression that is applied to the stomach with a sort of belt that is applied laparoscopically. This means that you do not need to have large incisions placed in you abdomen like before. Previously, there were much more radical approaches with open surgery done in a variety of ways. By employing the Lap Band procedure, surgeons have lessened the risks and lowered the costs.

But surgical approaches to weightloss are not for everyone. That's because they work so well that many people lose too much weight and then suffer from complications of malnutrition. I have found that there is a very nice dividing line between those who I feel are better off with Lap Band procedures and those who are better off with my own program. If you weigh less than 250 pounds as a woman or 300 pounds as a man, depending on your height and other factors, you are going to be able to achieve adequate results with my program in most cases. However, if you are over 350-400 pounds, you are most likely going to get better and faster results by taking the surgical approach. I am not saying that someone over 400 pounds cannot lose weight with my program. It's just that even if you lose 50-

100 pounds through my program, you are still going to suffer from significant obesity. For patients between 250 and 350, it is a case by case basis that determines which is better. Some will try my program first and base their decision on how they do with my program.

If you weigh less than 250 pounds, you may lose too much weight. I also have to deal with patients in my gynecology practice who suffer from hormonal aberrations due their excessive weightloss. A common problem is loss of menstruation because the body will not let a woman get pregnant if she is severely malnourished, so they do not ovulate. Lack of ovulation leads to lack of menstruation. Women who have had alterations in the function of the stomach are prone to vitamin, calcium, and iron deficiencies. The stomach secretes a chemical called Intrinsic Factor, which triggers the small intestine to absorb the Vitamin B 12. Thus we become concerned about Vitamin B12 deficiency after stomach surgery. Vitamin B12 deficiency is especially dangerous, leading to anemia and mental instability. One of my Obstetric patients had to actually gain 20 pounds before we could get her pregnant even with fertility pills. Now that she is pregnant, we are giving her injections with vitamin B12 and iron. She went into preterm labor and seem to respond best to an infusion of IV vitamins as a opposed to medications that we normally use to stop labor. She and I commiserate about what a shame it is that my program was not available when she was seeking treatment for weightloss. Nonetheless, she follows the progress of our weightloss program with great interest, because this is such a personally relevant subject.

Another issue with surgery is its permanence. With pills you can simply stop them and all of your body's survival adaptations return. This could be important if an asteroid hits earth. In a more practical scenario, you could find that you need the reserve to gain and maintain weight not only if you are pregnant but also if you were to get cancer. If you've had the gastric surgery, it could greatly interfere with your health as you go through chemotherapy.

The increased rate of weightloss also has its cosmetic issues. I have seen women lose as much as 30 pounds per month over the course of several months. With my program, a woman may at times lose over 22 pounds the first month, but I rarely see those kinds of results sustained beyond one month. Usually after the first month, the weightloss may fall so that ladies rarely lose more than an average of 15 pounds per month sustained over the first 3 months. A woman who goes from 260 pounds to 115 pounds in the course of a year will still have enough skin to cover a 260 pound body. Many women then have to follow up the weightloss surgery with multiple plastic surgeries to remove the baggy skin. By losing in smaller increments, my patients seem to have fewer issues with baggy skin.

The final issue is expense. These surgeries will usually cost at least $10,000. Sometimes there are bargains. Sometimes insurance programs will cover the cost. Including medication, my program should never exceed $200 per month and it can be as cheap as $120 if they can find bargains on the medicine. Thus, I do have many patients who would make good candidates for surgery who chose my program, because it's more affordable.

Finally, I do have some patients who have already had the surgeries, but over time, they have regained some weight. Now they seek me out to help them get some of the weight off. This is perfectly acceptable to me. Only now they can be where they need to be by losing less than 50 or 60 pounds rather than over 100. I have never combined Phentermine with surgery while the patient is in the initial year after surgery. I think a patient should wait and see how much they can lose on their own after the surgery before throwing medication into the equation.

I also want to add that it is possible to use the medication with other diet programs. My wife's ex-mother-in-law has decided to use my medicine with Nutri-Systems. She had previously used the low-carb diet with the pills, but she didn't like the low-carb. So now she has lost 14 pounds in the first month of her return to the program and she enjoys the meals. I never argue with success, but I do have issues with the concept that Nutri-Systems employs. They use the same argument to justify their approach as I use against it. They say that complex carbs sustains your blood sugar longer, which in turn keeps your appetite down. My argument against that approach is that you also do not burn fat when your sugar is up. Nonetheless, people achieve success here in as much as they still achieve some degree of control of portions. If you add in the Phentermine, you still burn calories faster and you won't find yourself snacking between meals either. Nutri-Systems provides your meals for you, thereby they control what you eat by feeding you. As long as you don't stray from their plan, they maintain the control. But like all diets, that's a big if. The cost is over $300 per month. My feeling is that if you are on the medication I provide, you shouldn't need a product like Nutri-Systems. Neither should you need a product like Weight-Watchers, Slim-Fast, or LA Weight Loss, but if you really want to incorporate any other program into you're your diet scheme, I'm not going to expend a lot of energy to try to talk you out of it. However, most of these programs are geared toward giving you a program with a dietary strategy to help you burn calories and control your appetite, whether it's through counseling, meal replacement products or supplements. With Phentermine, we accomplish both goals by lowering your appetite and causing your body to burn calories. Ultimately, the key is that you do something. In fact, we do offer some Physician's Weightloss products, such as some of their protein bars and shakes. However, I always emphasize that I don't want people to substitute other products for the medications that I recommend. Be that as it may, what you do when you leave the doctor's office is your own business. My attitude is that I work for you, not the other way around. If you find something that works for you, then my job is to help you get that approach to work best for you.

10

BurtmanWeightloss.com

I've already described how I initially became interested in developing what I've described as the Burtman Method of Weightloss. Now I want to update you on where we have gone with this program since I first started writing the book. I wrote my first words of this book at the end of 2005. I first started taking my own diet medications Thanksgiving of 2003. I placed my first advertisement for diet medications in April, 2004 in the Yellow Book. In about two years I had witnessed some awesome results. Thus, I undertook the writing of this book, because I thought that we were accomplishing great things through the program. Of course, there is nothing new or groundbreaking about what I suggest. It is the synthesis of several modalities and concepts combined into one method that has allowed us to be so much more successful than your basic diet pill supplier. There is no secret method by which I accomplish such profound weightloss in my patients. Any doctor can open his or her doors and offer exactly what I offer. As a physician, I thought that I should get the word out to allow other health care professionals and potential patients an opportunity to participate.

Now it's March 2008, and I'm still writing the book. I have written and completed 3 other books since 2003, and I have another half written. However, those books are all novels. I like writing novels. I admit it; carbohydrates aren't all that fascinating. I prefer writing stories. It's more entertaining for me to write good stories. So, this chapter will be sample of my story telling technique. Some will argue that this is some way for me to rationalize 2 ½ years of procrastination. I won't attempt to refute that; however, needless to say I've been a very busy guy, and I owe that fact largely to how successful we've been helping the people of Mississippi along with visitors from Alabama shrink.

We move now to Christmas of 2006. Rather than offering you the expected declarations of unparalleled success as a physician in Columbus, Mississippi, I have to instead inform you that I was on the brink of financial ruin. My primary job was as a fulltime Obstetrician and gynecologist. However, my workload was more suggestive of a part-time OB. My partner was and still is the hardest working OB in the world. As the relative newcomer to town, I was still struggling to build a large enough practice to maintain my financial commitments. At times I was quite busy and convinced that nothing could derail me, but suddenly in November, it was like someone had pulled a plug and the clinic seemed drained of patients. I had purchased other businesses that were also struggling, and the sudden downturn in revenue left me on the brink of bankruptcy.

At that time I begin looking for work elsewhere in Mississippi and the South at large. As I drove to some of my interviews, I had time to reflect on how I could implement changes in Columbus in terms of marketing what I had that was successful. With regard to weightloss, I realized that I still only had that one little Yellow Book ad that I had taken out as a favor to a friend in 2004. I also knew that we were coming up on peak season for people wanting to lose weight, New Years. I decided to run a series of business card size ads in our local newspaper. They commenced the week after Christmas. Within one week, I had gone from contemplating moving away to refusing any further interviews and turning down all job offers. We began seeing more patients than I had ever before seen in a day. By February, normally the shortest month and therefore the lowest revenue month for an office based practice, I had the most financially lucrative month of my life.

We had always used the traditional approach with my new weightloss patients. They were placed in a room just like any other appointment, and I went in and discussed my program individually with each person. It became terribly repetitious when I found myself saying the same thing 10 to 15 times a day, and I also found myself working until 6:30 every night. Then my nurse, Brandy, suggested that I talk to people in groups in my personal office from behind my desk just like we would in a seminar. With Brandy's suggestion, the light bulb went off. If I could see 5 or 6 at a time, why not more? I realized that the key component of my program was my counseling. There's no limit to how many people I can counsel at one time. Having been in the military, and having performed sports physicals for athletic teams, I also knew how to examine hundreds of kids of all ages quickly. If I could determine that a kid was fit to play football in a matter of seconds, I could determine that an adult was physically qualified to take diet pills in only seconds as well. The key was to be efficient while still being adequately thorough.

As we implemented this approach on a limited basis in the clinic, I began to envision a scenario where we took my show on the road. It also seemed a good fit with my personality. First, I like public speaking. I'm a ham and I admit it. I like attention and I like the idea of getting out there and having an impact on many lives in a positive way. I also joined a rock band in 2005, having just been taught how to play the bass guitar in a few months. Before long I was writing music of my own and then I purchased an old theater in Columbus called the Princess Theater in order to facilitate the development of my musical skills and career. The idea of incorporating my flair for the entertainment side of my interests would be an asset to developing the Burtman Weightloss road show. The other compelling thought was that if I could attract that many patients in a town of less 25,000, how many would I attract if I offered my services to people from more populated areas in Mississippi like Jackson and Hattiesburg. Furthermore, I was aided by the fact that there is still excessive fear and paranoia regarding diet pills throughout the medical field, despite the fact that I feel its based on preconceived notions that have no basis in fact or physiology. Nonetheless, I found myself with an unintentional monopoly on the diet pill business in Mississippi, because no other doctor offered diet pills on a large scale.

I joined services with a man named Chris Hannon whose background is in marketing and show promotion. We began devising a way to take our program on the road. We had folks driving all the way from Pascagoula, which is a 3-hour drive, just to get their diet pill prescription. Thus, we figured there would be a market throughout the state. We planned to offer a seminar that consisted of a 15 minute talk and a team of medical support staff to process the patients and take their vital signs. The patients were given medical questionnaires that allowed us to screen out those who were not medically qualified. Then I would go to every attendee and listen to their heart and lungs. This was the same way I could examine an entire squad of football players and medically qualify them for football. It was a matter of efficiency. The most important thing I do, besides writing the prescription, is the counseling. It didn't matter whether I was conversing with 5 people or 100. My workload would be the same either way. The major difference is that there was support both from my staff and from other people who attended the seminar, sharing their success stories. The only remaining issue was how to get the people to come and see us.

At first we took out ads in the newspaper. Our first seminar was attended by about 25 people in Tupelo, which is about 60 miles from us in Columbus. We also tried Granada, Hattiesburg, Meridian, and Jackson. In Meridian we only had 4 people. Needless to say, I was disappointed. However, we had another marketing idea that proved to be the smartest marketing ploy I have ever conceived of. I had grown my program in the office largely with word of mouth referrals. My patients lost 30 or 40 pounds and their friends couldn't help but notice. My patients became my walking billboards. Mississippi is the fattest state in America, so there was no shortage of eligible patients to take notice of their neighbor or family member losing weight quickly. Realizing that more of my patients came to me because they knew someone else on the plan, I decided to give back to those patients that recruited patients for us. I gave them $5 off for every referral. There was no limit to how many people they could refer. It only applied to the first visit, but it didn't take long for folks to realize that they could come for free if they brought us ten patients.

When numbers were down in Granada, Hattiesburg, Jackson and Meridian, we gave them an ultimatum: Deliver us at least 20 patients per seminar, or we would stop coming. We quit advertising, because people don't believe ads they see through the media. I can't blame them with so much BS out there on the airways and in print. But everyone believes their eyes when they see their friend drop 40 pounds in a matter of weeks to months. Of the preceding 4 towns, only Hattiesburg rose to the occasion. We were allowed to meet in a daycare center that was run by one of our patients. Nearly one year since their first seminar, I am proud to say that we outgrew the daycare and hosted 129 patients at a local hotel. That is our record as I am writing this now. Of course, as long as it is taking me to write this book, that record may be broken by the time I finish the book.

After the first few months of launching Burtman Weightloss, I began to think it wasn't worth the effort. The cost of advertising, gas, facilities, and staff was a financial drain. Notwithstanding the fact that I was wearing myself out with all of the driving, and I'm also a full time OB/GYN. I was about to call it quits on the whole seminar idea when I came up with another idea. I told my staff that I would give 20% of the proceeds to the coordinators for various locations. I now placed the responsibility in the hands of my coordinators for scheduling and recruiting of patients. Between the incentives for developing seminars given to my coordinators and the incentives to patients to find us other new patients, I suddenly discovered we were growing. We went from grandiose mass-market appeals to grass-roots face to face connections and it took hold over night. Instead of focusing on bigger cities, I let my staff find groups based largely on where they had contacts. My wife's cousin, Quintina Flake, knew people from all over the small towns in North Central Mississippi. So, having dropped larger towns like Jackson and Meridian, we established ourselves in smaller towns like Mathiston, Louisville, Starkville, and Forest. My own office nurse, Brandy Powell, found an alderman from a small town and arranged a seminar there. The town is called Vardaman. It is the sweet potato capital of the world. So guess what; lots of fat per capita. We have had over 100 people each of 4 months in a row. Brandy was angry to hear that Hattiesburg beat her record, so she hit the phones hard the next day trying to recruit enough patients to reclaim her record. And sure enough, there were 129 patients there. Unfortunately, one of them had a history of cardiac bypass surgery and was medically unqualified. This dropped Vardaman back to second at 128 patients. Still, I am quite pleased to have been informed that we drove the locale Weight-Watchers out of business. That leaves Monica Adams. She has been my most faithful coordinator, and she is a great fan of my rock band. She attended all of the early seminars when she got $50 for a long night that not only included working up overweight patients, but she also had to brave my driving from the back seat. Not only is she the coordinator of Hattiesburg and Tupelo, which are original locations. She also developed seminars in her hometown region of Amory and Smithville. We still meet in a home once a month in Smithville, but I'm afraid we are about to outgrow that country home in the middle of nowhere.

To say we were suddenly successful is an understatement. But then we became concerned that were too successful. Word of our prolific impact reached the Mississippi Board of Medical Examiners. They wanted to discuss my prescribing of diet medications in January of 2008. It was with great trepidation that we received this news. Was this to be the end of BurtmanWeightloss.com and our seminars? There were more far-reaching questions for me. I had to consider that my medical license might be in jeopardy. Everyone dependent on me and our program for income or treatment held their breath as the fateful day approached. I didn't know if this was indeed to be a discussion or an inquisition.

I arose early on January 14th for the drive to Jackson, unsure what awaited me there. Fortunately, it was cordial conversation designed to have a meeting of the minds, advise me of anything they didn't approve of, and satisfy their concerns that I was advocating lifestyle changes in addition to medication. Someone only needs to read this book or attend a seminar to know that my whole focus is on using the medication to change the way we eat. I was able to satisfy them that we were integrating the medication with counseling and denying medication to the medically unqualified, and we were allowed to continue. Now armed with board reviewed approval, we celebrated that night by seeing 106 patients in Vardaman.

Be The Least You Can Be

As I complete this chapter, I am now seeing enough success to actually consider quitting obstetrics to focus on weightloss. I enjoy it. It's fun to go into towns, entertain a little and provide a service that people truly appreciate. We still do most of our work in towns you can barely find on a map without the use of MapQuest. I can't help but wonder just how far this will go, but then again I don't want to put my whole future on the line with this either. There's a reason that most doctors in Mississippi won't prescribe these medicines. I still maintain its unadulterated fear with no basis in fact. However, in a trendy world, I can't completely base my career on diet pills. Eventually, there will be other doctors to see the light and offer competition. Maybe they will read this book and see the merits of this approach, or perhaps there will be some new innovation for weightloss. There will always be a need for birthing babies, and I hate to throw away the years of training that I endured to become an Obstetrician, but at the same time, there's still a lot of people in more populated areas than Columbus and Northern Mississippi that need my help. Time will tell, but all I know is we are still growing and no one else seems all that interested in providing this service, at least not here in Mississippi or Western Alabama.

11

THE BURTMAN METHOD OF LOSING WEIGHT IN A NUTSHELL

This is the nitty gritty. Just in case you don't want to read the whole book, here it is in its simplest form most condensed form.

Start the day off with a single dose of Phentermine. If not taken first thing, anytime in the morning is fine as long as it's before noon. Just remember the later you take it in the day, the later you are likely to stay up.

Eat two meals per day. I prefer to skip breakfast. It's your best opportunity to keep burning fat. It's also when you get the best therapeutic effects from the Phentermine, which makes breakfast the easiest meal to skip.

Take two Alli™ with every meal, or one Xenical if you are taking those instead. This will block the digestion of fat. One purpose in limiting you to two meals is to cut your cost with the Alli™/Xenical. Some people only eat one meal, simply because they are not that hungry. If that's you, then you need only take the Alli™ or Xenical once a day.

Remember that you will get hungry. Eating is still necessary for survival just like breathing and drinking. The difference now is that you can be satisfied with a low carbohydrate meal, meaning you won't need to stuff yourself with bread and potatoes to feel full. However, if you are not hungry, you do not need to eat in order to keep burning calories. The Phentermine is a stimulant that will keep you burning calories whether you eat or not.

You will be offered 6 prescriptions of Phentermine per year. You must be seen in person once per month to be weighed and checked before you will receive another prescription. The Alli™ is over the counter, so you can take that as long as you like. During the 6 months that you cannot take the Phentermine, you may be take Meridia and Strattera. I take both of them at lunchtime not on an empty stomach. Because they are not stimulants, you are given two refills with each prescription, so you only have to come once every 3 months if you wish to continue with these. They are better appetite suppressants than Phentermine, and they actually work better as you stay on them. They just cost a lot more and they don't rev up the metabolism the same way that Phentermine does.

The people who lose the most weight take both the Phentermine and Alli™ concurrently, and they come every month for 6 straight months instead of spacing out the prescriptions. The key is to use these medications to make the necessary changes in your eating habits to keep the weight off.

ABOUT THE AUTHOR

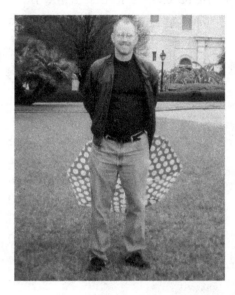

Mark Burtman is a board-certified physician, specializing in Obstetrics and Gynecology. He received his medical degree from Creighton University, in 1992.

Dr Burtman began his weight loss program in 2003 at his OB/GYN clinic in Columbus, Mississippi. His first patient was none other than himself. As his 40th birthday approached, he weighed 245 pounds, and he took 3 medications daily for the treatment of Type 2 Diabetes. It was time to do something. After researching the various options, he found the best combination of diet and medication, beginning on the Monday before Thanksgiving. In the first week he lost seven pounds. By Christmas he had lost eighteen pounds, and by the time he turned 40, in February, he had lost over thirty pounds. He has maintained his weight loss consistently since that time, and now only requires one medication per day, for his diabetes.

Inspired by his own success, he offered that same program to his patients. Soon, his patients' friends were coming to see him, after they saw the effectiveness of the program. That's when he purchased his first Yellow Book ad. Before long he was seeing 40-60 patients per month for his weight loss program.

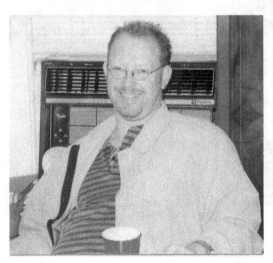

Since the first of the year, those numbers have grown to about 250 per month with 5-10 new patients added every day. Most of the new patients are referred by other patients. Why? Because this program works better than any other weight loss program in the country. "Having struggled with a weight problem of my own, believe me, if there was something better, I'd be doing it myself," says Dr Burtman.

Printed in the USA
CPSIA information can be obtained
at www.ICGtesting.com
LVHW042227301023
762626LV00004B/78